MW00962192

Gypsy Energy Secrets

Gypsy Energy Secrets

Turning a Bad Day into a Good Day No Matter What Life Throws at You

MILANA PEREPYOLKINA

This book is for informational purposes only and should not be used as a substitute for medical counseling with a health professional.
The author does not accept responsibility for such use.

Copyright © 2016 by Milana Perepyolkina
www.gypsyenergysecrets.com
All rights reserved.
No part of this book may be reproduced or transmitted in any form or by any means without written permission from Milana Perepyolkina.

Publisher's Cataloging-In-Publication Data
(Prepared by The Donohue Group, Inc.)

Names: Perepyolkina, Milana.
Title: Gypsy energy secrets : turning a bad day into a good day no matter what life throws at you / Milana Perepyolkina.
Description: North Charleston, South Carolina : CreateSpace Independent Publishing Platform, [2016]
Identifiers: LCCN 2016919280 | ISBN 9781539442257 | ISBN 153944225X
Subjects: LCSH: Attitude (Psychology) | Romanies--Social life and customs. | Romanies--Psychology. | Optimism. | Suffering. | BISAC: BODY, MIND & SPIRIT / New Thought. | SELF-HELP / Motivational & Inspirational.
Classification: LCC BF327 .P47 2016 (print) | LCC BF327 (ebook) | DDC 152.4--dc23

Printed in the United States of America

There is, I think in all women, a Wild and an Ancient Gypsy
who cries in anguish when we starch her flat.
There is a part of us that can never, ever be happy
until the Gypsy can Dance!
—Clarissa Pinkola Estes

Life isn't about waiting for the storm to pass…
It's about learning to dance in the rain.
— Anonymous (Let's imagine her as a wise old Gypsy woman)

Table of Contents

$\mathcal{O}ne$

RUNNING AWAY WITH THE GYPSIES

Something New Is Dancing

We all know heartbreak. We all know fear. We all know the feeling that we are not good enough. We feel the pain and anxiety of thinking we are alone, we experience that terrible worry that things may not work out for us. These fears are with us in many moments, but then something lifts us up out of darkness and into the light. It's always something simple that brings us joy—the feeling of the sun on our skin, laughter that comes from a deep place, the taste of something fresh and delicious, a strong hug from someone we know loves us very much. These are the things that call us home to ourselves.

I've recently come through a dark and difficult time, and so standing in the bright light of the sun and getting past fear and pain feels even richer to me now. That's the gift of a dark time—to show us the contrast of just how wonderful the light is and to deepen our gratitude for what we have.

"You're a *real* Gypsy?" the girl in a long skirt inquires loudly enough that a group of men and women gather around us. The intense blue sky illuminates the shimmering surface of white salt that stretches as far as the eye can see. We're surrounded by a landscape so flat we can see the curve of the earth, and our proper place on the planet is clear—we're insignificant, but also part of something majestic.

Salt has cleansing properties and is essential to supporting life. We are camping here on this bed of salt in this surreal place on an ancient lakebed on the Utah-Nevada border. We are experiencing things that will heal and cleanse us all in ways we can't even imagine yet. I know because I can smell it in the air that we will be forever changed by the time we leave this encampment.

I'm deeply moved that I'm considered a guest of honor here because I'm a *real Gypsy*! This means a great deal to me. More than the people gathered around me may realize.

Historically my people have been enslaved, feared, despised, and persecuted for who we are and what we know. Prejudice against Gypsies has been around for so long that many people who are careful not to be racist about other peoples haven't even questioned their negative beliefs about Gypsies—as if they are so true they don't need to be examined.

And now in the twenty-first century I'm here with over five thousand people on the Bonneville Salt Flats, and happy crowds are being drawn to me *because of* the Gypsy wisdom I freely share. I'm being treated with respect and even love by total strangers, not in spite of being a Gypsy, but because my heritage is now seen as making a valuable contribution here. I'm thrilled.

There are tents everywhere decorated with colorful fabric dancing in the powerful wind. The heat is intense, nearly unbearable. In this environment, water is not taken for granted. We can feel the moisture baking out of our bodies, and when fresh, cold, clear, clean water is passed between us it is a holy sacrament and nothing tastes better.

I'm surrounded by neo-Gypsies dressed in free-flowing clothes. They wear beautiful jewelry and scarves. Some think of themselves as bohemians or hippies. Those who claim the word "Gypsy" by affinity rather than birth are a loosely organized band of Americans who are living what they imagine is the Gypsy experience, some for just a few days, but others will fully embrace our way of seeing the world, and this will shape the rest of their lives.

There's music everywhere—inviting, intoxicating music. People dance in response. When we listen to the body and the body listens to music we sway and twirl because we must. I'm dancing to the call of the Gypsy spirit that runs through my ancient bloodline. I feel the joy of the dance! Letting go. Living fully. Why be the slave of our fears, limitations, and inhibitions? Life is such precious, beautiful thing, and it wants to be celebrated.

Dance. Connect with each other in the ways that matter, become one with the music, the land, the water, the sky, and the sun. We are one wild *taboro*, a word that means extended family. We are united, awakened, and aware. We are open to new experiences. We seek bliss as we dance and feel the music with every cell of our bodies. We experience life moving through us!

Everyone is excited to be here. I'm fully aware of how this emerging Gypsy movement can heal my people and so many others around the world. What was once despised is respected. What was put down is now elevated. The ancient knowledge we worked to keep secret and sacred for so long can now help guide modern life towards something better. Hundreds of thousands and even millions of people are discovering Gypsy wisdom and culture, and it is moving them to live fully—no matter what life throws at them.

People long to live with passion—in deep relationships that matter, in loving communities, in work that makes a difference, and to find powerful ways to cope with the realities of the world. They want to invite the deeper magic found in nature into their lives. This is our challenge as a global community of nations, families, and taboros—to see things as they really are and to be courageous about what it will take to address the problems we have caused in the world.

We long to find ways to celebrate in the midst of difficulty and to love ourselves and the natural world into complete balance and health.

In this colorful community gathered on the desert, men and women aren't just looking out for themselves, they are checking in with others to make sure food is shared, and to encourage each other to remember to drink water often in order to stay hydrated. I hear people comment that this level of caring for strangers is new to them. Gypsies take care of each other this way all the time, but think of how sadly rare it is to see this kind of loving concern among strangers demonstrated in a public way. Here in the desert it is essential that we look out for one another. I hope everyone takes this lesson home to environments that are more comfortable because we so desperately need real connection.

Our happy tribe has made things that are artful and useful, and those things are also being shared freely. The food is nutritious and fresh and is being passed around with generosity. I'm struck by how different this all feels from the "civilized" world back home. There are shows on television that claim to represent Gypsy life and that are so far from the "reality" I know that I can't even talk about them. The Gypsy family I've known all my life is an oasis of joy. The communities of Gypsies I know provide a safe haven away from the troubles of the world. Outside people who are not Gypsies may be angry and inconsiderate, but in the world of Gypsies many more people are warm and understanding. If I need help, everyone I know offers good advice and does what they can to help me. If someone is sick, everyone gathers to support them and their family.

If you are sad, everyone surrounds you to cheer you up. You are never alone, never forgotten, never left to struggle by yourself. We understand that sorrow that is shared becomes far less sorrowful and that joy that is shared becomes much more joyful.

Years ago when my daughter became sick with an illness that puzzled her doctors, I got on the phone and shared our family's struggle with just one call to one person, and a series of events were set in motion. Each one of my family members asked their friends and relatives, and a wide network searched for answers in books, in Gypsy practices, and in personal experience to solve the problem--immediately. Together, we found an answer and we healed her. I would never have been able to do that by myself. Everyone who helped was enriched by the experience. I knew my taboro had my back, and my daughter felt surrounded by love and support.

That's the kind of community this emerging Gypsy movement seeks to foster. I look around at the tents in the desert and see that people are expressing themselves much more freely and with louder laughter, bigger gestures, and much less inhibition than in the "regular" world. Strangers are immediately trusted. We look one another in the eyes and hold our gaze. Open hearts make it easier to quickly make real friends.

Someone is "telling fortunes" and I love seeing this because as advanced as we have become in the worlds of science and technology, we always want to know that there is a mystical element to our experience.

Something primal in us knows there are unseen worlds. And as soon as we inquire into these realms, they answer and give us support. I'm delighted that more and more science is proving the "unknowable."

Will there be an even stronger connection made between the mystical and metaphysical and the sciences in our lifetimes? Absolutely! And if it takes a bit longer that's fine. People will always follow their hearts, and their hearts will tell them divination has a place in their life experience. It always has and it always will.

We want to know that there is an underlying purpose to what happens to us. We want to know that we have a destiny or possibility that can be seen not just from where we stand at the moment, but at the edge of our experience in the way I can see the curve of the earth in the distance out here on the desert.

I stand in line with the others to see what this fortune-telling woman can offer about my own life. "What is foretold for me?" I inquire. "You have a very special gift for healing," she says, "and you must not hold it back any more. Share it with the world in the biggest way you can. You are safe. Give your talents freely. Be who you really are. Shine!"

As the sun sets I relax and disappear into the night sky for a long time. Without light interference from the city, the stars reveal themselves in much larger numbers and they seem bigger and brighter. In my imagination they wink at me. I play with them. I imagine that the stars love the fire we make in their honor. Fire dancers juggle fire sticks, spin fire hoops, twist fire chains, and play with danger. I see the courage in the people around me. Shine! Play with fire! What are you risking in order to experience more? The comfort of sitting on the couch doing nothing? Leaving the job you hate? Why not risk the things that don't matter for a chance to experience the things that do? Why not dare to do things we haven't tried before?

I recently wanted a new challenge, something that was out of my comfort zone, and so I taught myself to play the guitar. It wasn't easy. I wasn't good at it at first, but then after learning with passion and daring to be really bad at it and risking looking completely foolish, I finally clicked with my guitar, and now I love to sing songs I invent in the moment for myself and for others:

Darkness brings me happiness
In it I can sing and dream and dance
While no one watches
I can reach the stars
And shine so bright
That my light flies to your soul
And touches it

The conversations around the campfire are about how much fun it is to be in an unfamiliar place together, how great it feels to connect with nature, how fed up people are with the treadmill of life going nowhere—of working so hard for material things that don't even matter. People talk about how they want their families to be healthy, how they want to know their friends better, and how they don't want to be separated from each other anymore. They don't want to be slaves to dysfunctional institutions, gain the kind of education that doesn't enrich their lives, eat food that doesn't nourish their bodies, stagnate in marriages that offer no joy, move from relationship to relationship without healing anything, stagger around under debt, live in houses that are too big, drive cars that are too expensive, and waste years in jobs that aren't interesting enough or challenging enough to be worth the effort. "Everything we do has got to count. It's all got to be worth it!" I hear people share.

I love hearing the liveliness and the sense of demand these people express now. They will no longer tolerate a dull life. They will not plod along to the dreary end of life complaining all the way. Why don't more people make the choices that make it possible to live a long life that is deep and full of meaning?

I am asked many questions and there's so much to share that I feel that these days and nights on the desert are just the beginning. I do what I can to spark this desire for a holistic lifestyle and pray that it spreads like wildfire.

I teach people how to be resilient and joyful no matter what comes their way. I clap my hands under their noses to wake them up and I teach them what I know to inspire them to stop being spectators and to be creators! I look into the eyes of my brothers and sisters in the desert and say, "Life is outrageously spectacular! Don't settle for anything less!"

At the end of our time together as we tear down the camp, we take great care to make sure there is no impact from us having been there. We restore everything as it was. The only thing changed forever is that something new is dancing within us. What has happened in our hearts has made a fresh start. Our time together will make all the difference. This is a new beginning.

Where can we find you, our happiness?
Show us the path, show us the road

—Traditional Gypsy song

What Do You Know About Gypsies?

Juliette Binoche's character Vianne in the beautiful film *Chocolat* is a nomadic single mother of Gypsy heritage. She carries on the ancient tradition of dispensing remedies for the body and soul using her intuition about what each person needs. She is happily seduced by Johnny Depp's character Roux when he arrives in her French village with his band of Gypsies, and along the way the audience is also seduced by what these two embody of the Gypsy soul.

Vianne understands that she is in charge of her enjoyment of life, and that this pleasure doesn't depend on her circumstances but on her capacity for joy and her personal courage in the face of life's difficulties.

She shows us that loving life in all its messiness is a very desirable quality. People are universally drawn to the quality of courage. This passion for living comes from knowing life is short and that we must take risks and be bold in order to live fully. Escaping and disappearing into a comfort zone is a deadly place to be and will lead to an incomplete and short life if we surrender to the ordinary.

Feeling excitement for your life *as it really is* in all its painful and messy reality feels much different than having a fantasy about what life should be and complaining about what you don't have and don't experience. Becoming grounded and being real is at the center of creating something powerful. We say we don't want hard times, but there's a deep confidence that comes from surviving difficult times by being resourceful, inventive, and resilient.

When you live authentically, including suffering authentically and celebrating authentically, you sing with a full voice.

When you know you can overcome anything, this self-reliance settles in your bones and you are free to dance your way through life.

When you know how to find peace in chaos, you can greet whatever happens with open arms.

I'm here to show you how to master the art of going *without* something you really don't need. I'll show you how to make do with *what you have* with a deep sense of gratitude. I'll help you explore the ways you can find the *freedom to appreciate your life* and the people, animals, and things in it. I'll show you how to call abundance and love into being. And I'll show you how to find strength even when you are depleted, so that you can be a truly powerful and magical person.

What do you think you know about Gypsies? Many people know only the tired old stereotype that Gypsies read fortunes and steal chickens. My people have been known to fill a pot with meat unknowingly donated by a farmer somewhere. But let's be fair and honest about this. There are plenty of well-educated, established people who have been known to commit immoral actions, whether it be cheating a few millions here and there or engaging in acts of severe discrimination. Yet that behavior doesn't indict an entire race or class of people—does it? The morally wrong actions of some do not define the group from which they come. Bad or good behavior doesn't have anything to do with being a Gypsy or non-Gypsy, it's an individual choice of how to live and interact with others. We'll leave unethical people from all communities to face the consequences of their poor choices. They can do what they want. We will chose to live our way. Choose well and good things will be drawn to you.

Another image of Gypsies comes from reality television shows that take a tabloid approach to showing the extreme behavior of a very few people as representing an entire culture. They were chosen for the series because of their extreme behavior. They are not the norm. These shows reinforce ignorance about and prejudice towards Gypsies and may seem to be authoritative on the subject, but in reality they are just a mishmash of dysfunction wrapped up in sensationalism and not about anything of substance.

If you're curious about the *real* experience of Gypsy people who honor their culture around the world and are good people doing good things, there do exist some very good books and films. There's a fine documentary that follows three Gypsy children in Romania and explores the segregation and isolation they face and also what they are doing to create a better life. *Our School* is intelligent, beautiful, and worth seeing. I would also recommend the book *We are the Romani people* by Ian Hancock if you'd like to learn the history of my people. *Romani* is the right word for people known to the Western world as Gypsies.

There's much to explore if you're curious about real Gypsy culture. What I'm going to share with you in the pages of this book is old and respected Gypsy wisdom that has great integrity and is steeped in tradition and magic. It comes from ancient traditions that have been cultivated and protected over time. I'll show you a way of living that has endured in spite of many attempts to eradicate it, including the extermination of Gypsies by the Nazis.

The Gypsy way of being is a rich and vibrant tradition that continues to thrive in many places around the world, even though there is ongoing discrimination against the Romani people in many places. Gypsies continue to suffer rejection and harsh treatment. They endure violations of their human rights. Many lack medical care, housing, and education. Even now Romani people face employment discrimination and violence. In well-developed countries with progressive views about just about everything else, it is still seen as acceptable to discriminate against Gypsies. But in spite of this, Gypsies carry on dancing and singing and living life fully and with passion. My encouragement to you is this: if the Romani can live well under these difficult circumstances, know that you too can thrive in your life right here, right now!

Do you face financial stress that grinds you down? Do you worry too much, focus on the negative too often, experience life as drudgery except for those rare times when you have a vacation? Is your mood too dark and your energy flat? Does your body lack vibrant, good health? Do you struggle to balance the demands of family and work and drop exhausted into bed after watching television because there isn't much left of you at the end of the day?

Gypsy wisdom will help you become more capable, vital, grounded, healthy, and joyful. You'll have more to offer yourself, your family, your community, and the world. I promise that if you nurture a part of you that can become your inner Gypsy, life will be better. Trust me. I've helped many people live well and am able to see into the future from time to time. Let's make certain that your future unfolds as you wish.

A Very Short Story of A Long Journey

The written record of Gypsies is often found in the records of those who dominated our people, so hear this short tale of our past with that understanding. Gypsies began moving from India to other places in the world in about the tenth century A.D. In India, male Romanies were often craftsmen for royal families, and female Romanies entertained royal families with their singing and dancing. Two thousand years ago, Indian royal families frequently rose and fell in power because of constant wars between them. Many Gypsies suffered as slaves. They moved from one royal palace to another until they began an exodus out of the region, one group at a time. They reached Byzantium in the twelfth century and Western Europe in the fifteenth century.

When asked where they came from, Gypsies sometimes said, "From Little Egypt." Little Egypt was a province in Byzantium. The English word "Gypsy" came from the word "Egyptian." But people in most European countries used variations of the word "Atsingani" to name Gypsies. In Russian, "Tsygane," in German "Zigeuner," and in French "Tsigane." The word "Tsygane" is not used by most Romanies because of its association with hundreds of years of slavery.

The spiritual roots of our culture are similar to the Atsingani who were members of a religious group known for its magical powers. Atsingani were said to be the descendants of Simon Magus, or Simon the Sorcerer. Simon lived two thousand years ago in Samaria. It was said that he could perform miracles that the apostles could not and he gathered large followings in every city he visited. Legend has it that people were astounded by his ability to heal and perform wonders such as standing unharmed in fire, making bread from stones, traveling through the air, causing objects to move, and opening locked doors without touching them.

During the same time period, in the same area, both Simon and Jesus performed miracles, provided healing, and were described by Romans as *magicians,* which had a different connotation at the time than the word has now. Both had big crowds of followers. Both were killed by people whose religious beliefs were threatened by them and the freedom they tried to offer people. Simon was stoned to death and Jesus was crucified. We don't know much about Simon because his followers were peaceful and didn't use the force of arms to spread their religion. When the Christian church shifted from being a prosecuted minority to becoming organized and powerful, anyone associated with the teachings of Simon Magnus was automatically accused of being connected with the devil.

It was said that the marvels Simon had performed were witnessed by so many that the early fathers of the Christian church made no attempt to deny them. They could only argue that since such things should rightly be done only in the name of Jesus, Simon must be in league with the devil, which he was not. He stood in opposition to harmful forces and in favor of the light and the good. But because he and his followers didn't join the early fathers of Christianity they branded him as coming from a dark place. Many of the teachings collected by his supporters were burned and his followers were killed. There were many attempts to eradicate this culture and only a very few texts are left that allow us a glimpse into Simon's teachings.

Simon Magus taught that Fire is One Power and the source of all that is—the seen and unseen. Fire has a central place of importance in the lives of Gypsies. Simon's teachings included the Tree of Life or the Cosmic Tree—the underlying structure of everything and the way we are connected above and below. Simon Magus was said to fly through the air, and Gypsies came to believe that they had once flown through the air like birds. Simon Magus taught about three Worlds: the Divine, Middle, and Lower. This has a parallel with the traditional Gypsy teaching about the Upper, Middle, and Lower Spiritual Worlds.

Did Gypsies use the same "source" of wisdom and power as Simon Magus? And where did their beliefs originate? Gypsy women predicted the future and were both feared and sought out for their ability to cast a positive spell or to throw a curse. Gypsy men tamed bears and healed horses. All Gypsies had a vast knowledge about healing herbs and rituals. They could create a magical talisman that would bring good luck.

Gypsies were seen as being connected to some kind of magic, but this was only documented in written records when Gypsies finally reached Europe because their wisdom had only been passed in oral tradition before that point. By the time anything about Gypsy culture was written down, it was being written by the people who stigmatized, controlled, and feared Gypsies.

Throughout this book I will use the words "Gypsy" and "Gypsies" because most readers are familiar with them, but I also want to introduce you to the proper terms "Romani" and "Romanies", and I will sometimes use the word "Roma" because it is used in several Romani dialects. Romanies don't really like to be called Gypsies because the word is connected with negative stereotypes and discrimination and was a word chosen by the people who dominated us.

Now that you know the short history of Gypsies you'll be able to call my people by their proper names and share their origin story in a kinder way than is usually told.

I want to point out from the beginning that this book does not represent the views of all Romanies—the traditions of different Romani nations vary a great deal. I can only share with you what I know from the Russian Romani, *Russka Roma*, point of view because that is what I was taught. However, all Romani nations celebrate and share something in common from our historical and mythical origins and our lives in the modern world—we share a tradition of being deeply connected to nature.

As Romanies traveled the world, we gathered a wealth of natural healing techniques from every culture and refined and honed those that were the most effective. In order to survive under harsh oppression, we learned how to communicate with all parts of nature, the seen and the unseen. I will guide you to follow the footsteps of the Romanies, and you too will learn some of the magic of the seen and unseen.

*   *   *

I've been called a healer, but I don't believe that I do the healing, so I look for another way to describe what I do. The body heals itself much of the time when given the right support. I have practiced the collected wisdom of my family and my people and I have studied with powerful healers, learning and testing what works and sifting through the wisdom of the ages. I am not a doctor. I do not diagnose or treat disease. But I believe that there is one road to true and complete health, no matter what the disease or illness, and that this path is available to all of us.

Romanies use different words for *doctor* in the twenty-five major Romani nations—each nation in a different territory of the world and each speaking a different language or dialect.

In Welsh Romanes (the Romani language spoken in England in a place dominated by Western medicine) the word for "doctor" is *drabengero*, from the word *drab* which means poison. So, *drabengero* is literally a man of poison.

In Russian Romanes (the Romani language spoken in places where alternative medicine is very popular) the word for "doctor" is *sastipnari*, from *sastipen* which means "health."

The Russian word for health is *zdorovie*, from the word *zdorovo* which means fine or great. A healthy person does feel great. The Romani word for healthy is *sasto*, close to *sastir* meaning iron. It is interesting that Russians say about someone who has exceptional health, "This person has iron health."

Gypsies living in Russia absorbed that language and culture, and so the word for a healer is *tselitel*, from *tselyi* which means whole. So, *to heal* is *to make whole*. The Romani word for "to heal" is *mendini*, very close to the English word mend. One of the meanings is "to restore to health."

I like to describe myself with a word I created to reflect what I do. I say "healther" in English. The word *healther* comes from combining the words helper and health, meaning a health maker. I help people become healthy again by providing them with the Gypsy map to the road of health. Are you intrigued? Are you open to receiving the gift of this way of being? Are you willing to explore? Will you be brave about taking on a few new ideas to see if they are a fit for you? Then let's begin.

Discovering Gypsy Magic

This book will help you celebrate life and cultivate the ability to find the good in your experiences, no matter what. This is the special wisdom that has helped the Roma survive when the entire world was against them. When someone has nothing, is sick, mistreated, and there is no help on the way–what can be done? As it happens, there is a great deal that can be done. One open and lively smile, eating something wonderfully nutritious, and focusing on something, anything that will bring a ray of hope, are all abundant riches.

I've been through extremely miserable and difficult times in my life, and I consciously chose to focus on one or two things that could get me through the worst of my days.

I find great inspiration in the Romani way—being bold, passionate, and full of energy. Here is just one thing we know that can shift your perspective. We know how to dance when we are miserable and when we are happy. When was the last time you really danced? Not at a nightclub or a wedding. Not feeling self-conscious about how you looked or trying to impress. I mean dance from the inside out. Dancing is not only for a rare and special occasion like a big night out or a celebration. Dancing is for everyday! Dancing is for when you cannot stand the pain of life one more minute. Have you ever danced when you were sad? Have you ever danced when you were angry or hurt? Have you ever thrown your head back and stomped your feet?

Promise me that you will try this the next time you are ecstatic, in despair, or feel hurt or hopeless. Promise me that you will experiment with the ideas in this book, not just in your head as you read, but by actually *doing* with your body what you read so that you have the physical experience of Gypsy magic. Will you dance today? At the beginning of our journey together, will you dance just to begin to get a feel for this? Pick music you know will make you want to move and set yourself free. Notice what comes up. Notice any discomfort. Push through it. To be *free* takes effort.

I think it is unfortunate that for many people life is too normal, too good, too comfortable. Most people are inclined towards too much of a good thing, which turns out to be very bad for you.

What passes for normal life is eating food that tastes good but is not nutritious, tolerating a job and liking it just enough to be trapped by it and therefore not being called to your true vocation. Having a family but not treasuring the gift of your family. Being in a relationship but not being passionate about your relationship. Being in a community of some kind, but not really investing yourself in building and enhancing it.

People commonly have the problem of having too much that doesn't mean much and not having enough of the important things that really feed the soul. They are not satisfied but are complacent and inactive and don't take their life head on.

There is a tendency to absorb too much passive entertainment that really isn't very entertaining or useful, and after a while we become so desensitized that we no longer discriminate about what we take into our lives.

We lose our ability to be demanding. We lose the ability to say *no! Damn it NO!* powerfully and passionately when something is wrong for us, and to embrace *yes! I say YES!* when we know something is right for us.

When people get sick, they take pills rather than try to get to the root of the sickness. They tolerate "temporary relief" as you see on the bottle of many "medicines," rather than the real relief that takes more work and more struggle but provides the lasting benefit of robust health.

When people get sad, angry, or depressed, they don't grieve and wail and scream and get it out of their bodies. When they are angry, they do not shake their bodies and listen to what it is they really need and demand and claim what they want. When they are dissatisfied, they don't act bravely to take a risk and change their lives.

What is too much and what is too little? A real Gypsy who knows their cultural tradition and has respect for it can tell you that there is wisdom in the idea of moderation in all things, including moderation. An occasional "too much" of something can be a celebration that is good for the heart. Drinking at a gathering can be just the right thing for the soul. Even drinking a little too much once in a while can be just right to cause a breakthrough. But taking drugs or drinking alcohol unconsciously, every day, every week, every month to numb the pain that you don't dare feel or to artificially generate the excitement that is lacking in your life, or to temporarily lower inhibitions but not really dismantle them, will not make you feel safer, more joyful, or truly *alive*. Numbing yourself will kill you slowly and will drain the passion from your life. There is "spirit" in substances, but it can distract you from connecting with a deeper kind of spirit, so be very cautious.

There is a way to experience a higher state of freedom, wholeheartedness, and a heightened way of living without alcohol or drugs. Only what is *real* and grounded and healthy will feel real to your soul.

The truth has always been with us but has often been withheld. I share Gypsy energy secrets with you now because I believe that the mysteries of well-being need to be given much more freely than they have been in the past. For too long things that were sacred were held closely by a few people who wanted to use what they knew to exercise power over others. The time for people to control information to gain power or to be greedy about secret knowledge is over.

This is a time when good ideas about the health of our bodies, spirits, and the planet need to be shared with all of the human family. We need each other to survive and thrive. We are all neighbors in this global community. We are one human family—all branches of the same cosmic tree.

I will share with you what I know about health, resilience, and well-being with the understanding that there is more wisdom to come. There is an old Gypsy saying, "Live one hundred years, learn one hundred years, and yet at the end, you'll still know nothing." Remember that.

I continue to learn from other healers in a spirit of humility, and I encourage you to join me on this journey of knowing and not knowing. Are you ready to receive? Are you willing to try things that may be new to you? Will you risk something to gain something greater?

There is a Gypsy legend that from the very beginning of time the secrets of the Kingdom were compiled into one book by God. This book had no words. It was made of cards with pictures and symbols on them. The Devil tried to steal these cards from God. The Devil wanted them only for himself and wanted to keep their divine power away from the people of the Earth, but as he stole them he dropped them and they rained down from the sky and blew in the wind all over the world. Everyone was asleep except the Gypsies, who were up singing and dancing by the fire. They saw the cards falling from the sky and decided to put the book God had made back together. So, they began traveling from place to place in search of the lost cards. They found the cards that taught them how to read a person's future. They found the cards that allowed them to look at each person's past to offer them more understanding of the present. They found the cards that taught them how to communicate with nature. Still, many cards were missing and so the Gypsies kept moving from place to place in search of every piece of wisdom that had been scattered. To this day Roma say, "Cards know the truth by themselves because they come directly from God."

Two Sides of One Coin

Ask me who I am and I will tell you that long before I was born, fate brought two people together who would marry magic and science in an unusual way. My great-grandmother was a wise and intuitive Gypsy and my great-grandfather was a Russian doctor with a scientific mind. I feel this inheritance intertwined in my soul—my Gypsy and Russian soul that loves both the rational and the mystical.

When I was a child growing up in Estonia, I was captivated by the Gypsy culture surrounding me. I grew up hearing the music of tambourines and guitars. I admired the glitter of chandelier earrings and the dramatic sweep of long, brightly printed skirts. My world was full of strong flavors and many bright colors, and I rode horses from the time I was very young. The horses were full of spirit and I was encouraged to be spirited too. I learned traditional Gypsy songs like this one:

Horses were taking the Gypsies away
City lights shining, ending the day
Oh how I long to join you in my mind
My soul's sorrows leaving behind

In those glorious days of freedom, I was allowed to get dirty and fall down and make mistakes. Adults seemed to be looking the other way so that we children could experience some level of danger and really live. I was free to try things and succeed and fail. I was encouraged to be independent and to explore.

I loved the company of people who saw their experience as an endless journey without a destination. I loved wearing the traditional Gypsy dress and dancing, dancing, dancing.

When Gypsies dance, we hold our heads high, our arms move with the confidence of a bird's wings in flight, and our feet trick the eye into thinking that we are gliding just above the floor, and then we land--with powerful stomps of our bare feet. We clap and shout out encouragement to each other. We are a noisy, vibrant, and joyful people.

From the time I was young I loved to hear and tell stories. The other children would gather around me in a circle and I would tell them story after story. I shared things I had heard from my parents and grandparents. When I finished, the children would call out, "Tell us more! Tell us more!"

Life was harder when we had to live in a densely populated apartment block in a big city. I was still a girl, but I was the only fortune-teller in my neighborhood. In this setting my parents and I had to hide our Gypsy identity because it wouldn't have been safe. If a woman told fortunes, she could be punished. Anything to do with spirituality or magic was illegal, although some brave Gypsies women did take the risk. They would position a lookout at outdoor markets and train stations—someone who would whistle a warning if the police approached—and would tell fortunes and read palms. In doing this they were at risk for being beaten, arrested, and put in prison.

During the warm months, the children of the neighborhood gathered on a grassy field between the towering apartment buildings to hang the washing that had been done in bathtubs. We lugged the wet laundry down the flights of stairs in big baskets and hung it out to dry on long lines in the sun.

We had other chores as well, including beating rugs thrown over tall poles with sticks until no more dust flew out of them. When our work was done, I used cards and palmistry and provided my intuition about the young lives of my friends. I was right much more often than I was wrong, and this built my confidence in my intuitive gifts. "I see you have this particular wish that you'd like to come true" I would share, and I would somehow know what that was in great particular. "Look, you are presently right here (I would point to an area on the palm), in the land where wishes do not come true no matter how hard you want something. And here (I would point at a different spot) is the place where your wish can come true. What you need are the directions to get from here to there." Then I would use the cards to find out which steps had to be taken in order for the wish to come true. My friends thought I had supernatural powers. Somehow I just knew what to say and that it wasn't me saying it but a wisdom coming through me that was meant to be useful and helpful in the growth of the person in front of me. Because I could see and hear what had the potential to be, I could help provide the guidance to what was possible if the right steps were taken.

I think I had this clarity because I lived a small part of the year freely in nature. I rode horses, communicated with the Earth, and experienced the power of my own soul in connection with nature. I had the confidence to say what I knew to be true, even at a young age.

I already knew my "supernatural powers" came from a source that traditionally sustained Gypsies for hundreds of years—a connection to the energy of the Earth. From the time I was four until I was fifteen, I spent each summer at a camp far away from the city in a forest next to the Baltic Sea. This camp had no plumbing or hot water. I would take off my shoes and walk everywhere barefoot. I would sit on the ground, play on the ground, and sleep on the ground. I would climb a tree and sit on one of the top branches becoming one with that big, tall, wise old tree, feeling and receiving love. I would not make a sound. I would even breathe as quietly as I could and I would not move so I could feel the connection. I would just look, listen, and connect. I would observe birds and squirrels from my little throne in the Kingdom of the World and talk to them with my thoughts. I knew when my thoughts were getting through to them, because they would come near and speak in their own particular language to me. It was a language without words, and it was a sacred and beautiful thing to be understood by the animals and to be able to understand them as well.

When I'd had my fill of time in the trees, I would climb down and run to the beach. I'd put warm, white sand into my palms and gently blow on it, looking at the patterns the little grains of sand would make. Each summer, I was connected to nature in this very profound way and that sustained and nurtured me.

Parents were only allowed to visit the camp once a month for a few hours. And how wonderful it was that the counselors—only one for every forty children!—left us pretty much to ourselves. I could go anywhere in the forest by myself and spend hours feeling at one with the trees, the animals, the stars, the waves of the sea, the wind, and all parts of nature. I was able to experience the Kingdom, which is how we Gypsies experience the natural world. It was my playground and I was the plaything of the Universe. But with all the joy I experienced in nature, there was also a great deal of darkness in my world.

The former Soviet Union was a very harsh place in which to live. It was a place where Gypsies and others who stepped outside of the boundaries narrowly defined by the government were punished severely. I had an uncle who was sent to prison for owning an unsanctioned book about healing that was found in his apartment by the authorities. People who were picked up disappeared, and many were never heard from again.

My mother worked in an office where at the end of long days she was required to stay into the evening to hear stern lectures about the superiority of the Soviet system, and she was forced to speak in front of others about the importance of strict atheism, even though she had a much more magical and spiritual view of the world and her place in it. Being forced to tell those lies hurt her body and her soul deeply. I watched how difficult it was for her to betray her most authentic way of being—it made her heartsick and it made her physically sick as well.

When we lived in the city we had the poorest quality of canned and dried food, and there was no variety in our diet. We also had poor quality water. We went without fresh produce most of the year, enjoying living food for only a few weeks out of twelve months. We were all sick, undernourished, or unhealthy in some way or another, and our souls suffered.

I learned from the adults around me that I had to be very careful about being a Romani. I learned that I must make my fortune-telling something of a game or a joke, because if I, or others, appeared to take it seriously, I would be in a dangerous position and may be locked away in a psychiatric hospital. So I grew up having two very distinctly different experiences that have prepared me for my life work as a healer. I know what it is like to be utterly free and full of robust health, and I know what it is like to be controlled, diminished, and unhealthy. I am glad for this dual experience because it gives me a compassionate point of reference when I help people live a healthy life.

From early childhood, I learned ancient healing techniques and remedies from my family. My father was *shuvihano*, which means a keeper of secret knowledge. My mother and father were divorced when I was young, and when I visited my father he told me beautiful folk tales and shared the wisdom of natural healing with me. My mother also used traditional Gypsy healing techniques when there was no doctor, and even sometimes when a doctor was available, she thought the medicine would do more harm than good.

I watched in awe as my grandmother confidently saved my cousin's life after a drowning accident by quickly tapping a few needles into key energy points of his body. He went from being still and blue to expelling the water from his lungs and rising up alive and well in my grandmother's arms.

These ancient techniques are based on a deep knowledge of the energy exchange that goes on between human beings and the Kingdom of the World—which is how Gypsies think of the natural world. These practices don't separate a human being from nature, but rather connect us to it more lovingly and more powerfully.

These Gypsy ways of living stand in sharp contrast to the clinical version of modern medicine, which looks at a person's body not only as separate from nature, but also at different parts of the body as being separate from each other. For traditional Gypsy healers, such an approach is nothing short of crazy!

I understand that a level of specialization is useful in negotiating the complexities of modern medicine, but it can also be unintentionally harmful when doctors and patients forget to pay attention to what it takes to truly heal the entire body and the soul.

To be whole we must work with the connections between all parts of the body, the physical body and the spirit, the person and their family and friends, and the natural world around them. That is complete medicine. That is the real source of healing.

When I was sick as a child, my mother would have a doctor diagnose me—because I had to get a doctor's note in order to be excused from school—but after the doctor handed over the note and medicine prescription it seemed as if my mother couldn't wait to close the door and teach me the traditional healing technique for whatever ailed me. Unfortunately, I was a rebellious child. At the time, I didn't want to follow my parents' old fashioned healing methods because they seemed irrational, and I wanted to be someone who was sophisticated and modern and logical.

So I've had the life experience of both valuing and devaluing my Gypsy heritage at different times in my life, and this has also prepared me for facing the harsh judgments about Romanies that I've heard from other people. I had those judgments myself for a period of time, so I understand. This range of experience has also helped me resolve my own internal dialogue about traditional wisdom—which I have come to embrace with all my heart.

Everything I know about the ancient energy work and healing techniques of the Romani was learned and then refined by practical application. I have integrated what I know by passing on what I have learned.

After my father died I decided it was time to preserve this knowledge by writing it down for my daughter. It was when I began to write with the intention of preserving Gypsy wisdom for my own family that the two parts of my soul began to fight again.

The Russian soul is known for its openness. When you meet a Russian stranger, within ten minutes he will have shared his deepest desires and biggest problems. On the other side of the coin, the Romani soul is closed to *gadje* (outsiders, non-Romanies) because so often the Romani have been discriminated against. Roma say, "With outsiders, play hide-and-seek and in puzzles you must speak." You may live next door to a Gypsy family for years and never know anything about them. If you meet a Rom (male Romani) on a street and ask his name, he will tell you a name straight away, although it may not be his *real* name. It may be a random name he picked in order to hide his real identity, not necessarily because he himself is untrustworthy, but because he does not trust *you* yet.

The Russian soul is shared freely and the Gypsy soul is a puzzle under lock and key. Russian poetry and language is full of the exquisite suffering and joy of life with the soul bared to the reader. In the Romani community, the practices of a *shuvihano* are never written down and thinking about publishing them is in itself taboo. Also, the Romanies didn't have a written language for a thousand years and only during the last one hundred years have books become widely available in the Romani language. An additional complication to sharing our traditions is that Russian Roma use the Cyrillic alphabet and European and American Romanies use the Latin alphabet. So you see, it's even hard for us to share our wisdom amongst ourselves around the world!

I have faced a dilemma about how much of what I have written as a record for my family I should share with you, and what I should keep for myself and my people. In the end, I feel good about my choices in this regard. In the pages of this particular book, you will read about some methods that are no longer commonly practiced by some communities of Romani people. Many traditions have almost been lost because they were not preserved well or passed down to the next generation. Some of the practices I share in the book may be unique to my family lineage. Some ideas are coded for outsiders, but Romani readers will be able to read more between the lines.

As with any traditional wisdom, you need to understand that a teaching that can be used in a positive way can also be employed in a negative and dark way to cause harm. I *never* go to those places and I strongly recommend that you don't either. Our energy is too precious to be wasted on anything that is harmful to ourselves or others.

Always strive to act with a kind and loving heart and in ways that are in tune with the loving energy of the Kingdom of Nature, and your life will bring healing benefit to the entire planet and make your own life magical.

Dictionaries define "magic" as either the use of charms or spells believed to have supernatural power over natural forces, or extraordinary power or influence seemingly from a supernatural force.

Gypsies know that *magic* is the extraordinary power that comes from knowing how to communicate with the force that orders the Universe, with nature, and with the sacred energy that holds everything in balance.

Practicing the magic of life does not make anyone superior to Nature, it is enough to be in harmony with it. When you are in balance you will experience a grounded and extraordinary sense of natural power.

I heard this story when I was a young child from my great-great-grandfather, who heard it from his great-great-grandfather who swore that this story was true. It happened a very long time ago. How long ago you ask? If you could travel back in time, it would take as long as it would for a bird to fly to the Sun. Back then Gypsies had wings. They could fly anywhere they wished. They would rise above the Earth and admire Her wonders the silvery threads of rivers, endless pastures, solemn mountains, and playful seas. Our people flew anywhere their souls' desires took them and things were easy perhaps too easy. One day, Gypsies were flying high above the Earth and saw wild horses galloping over the surface of the Earth. The Gypsy people could not take their eyes off the graceful and powerful horses turning together with their hooves thundering and moving so beautifully in a way that was very much connected to the Earth. The Gypsies talked amongst themselves and decided to ask God to exchange their wings for horses. Said-and-done. God took their wings and the Gypsies descended to the Earth to live on the ground but with the freedom that comes on the back of a horse. From that time forward, horses were our best friends. We say, Gypsy and a horse have one heart.

When I talk about the Kingdom, I mean "everything that is." Some people refer to *it* as God, some call *it* nature. I also like to use the word "Universe" because it includes all forces, seen and unseen.

When I need help, I call upon my own intuition and the power of the wind. I may ask my ancestors for help, or I may address the whole Universe for assistance.

I personally believe this is what a certain kind of spirituality is really about: accepting that there are different types of forces that were created to help us and to connect with all of them through love and gratitude.

It's not important which word you use to name "everything that is" or how you address the higher unseen forces or force around you. What is important is that you acknowledge that there is something wise and loving out there and that whatever it is, it is directly available to *you*.

When you ask a question, you may not know exactly what it is that answers you. What is important is that you learn how to hear the answer and use this communication to create a magnificent reality for yourself.

There are not many spells or charms in this book. One should be extremely careful with any kind of spell because something can easily go wrong. I've been practicing magic for a long time, but I still made a mistake of purpose and intention that taught me that important lesson.

One summer night, I was awakened by a very demanding white-bellied-blacked-tailed bird. This magpie decided to chat obnoxiously right next to my bedroom window. I looked at my clock; it was only five in the morning. The magpie would not stay silent for the next three hours, although I asked her to leave several times. The next morning, it happened again. I firmly asked her to leave. She didn't. After a sleep-deprived week I decided to put a spell on her. I got so angry that I thoughtlessly cast a spell to silence her, instead of a spell to just get her to move on. The morning after the spell was blessedly quiet and I was happy about that, until I found the dead magpie in my backyard. I was devastated. I didn't want the chatty bird to be silent in this particular way; I just wanted her to move to a different place, but that wasn't the intention I sent out into the Universe. It was the first time a spell did not turn out the way I expected, but it was enough to stop me from using spells for a while. Now each time I see a magpie, I ask for forgiveness. I think I will be doing this for the rest of my life. Keep this story in mind when you will be practicing spells. Follow my guidelines word-for-word. I will offer you sacred rituals that do no harm because I have learned from my mistakes.

I have prayed throughout the making of this book that it will offer you comfort, a safe haven, and experiences that are useful to you living a great life. Open it when you feel sad, lonely, hurt, or when you are at a crossroads and are wondering how to act. I have written this book to show you how you can find a state of quiet happiness, the kind where a smile barely touches your lips and yet your eyes are filled with light.

I have written this book to help you feel yourself open up to new possibilities, to imagine that your soul is a beautiful flower that you are tending to so that it will fully bloom. I pray that you will feel like the sun, shining with brilliant light, giving out warmth and love, and accepting whatever life throws at you with poise, dignity, and gratitude.

I feel blessed by the opportunity to help preserve a rich and uplifting aspect of my heritage that is in danger of being overlooked or erased and to show you the magical side of the Kingdom of the World.

Two

Connecting With The Kingdom

God is in the Forest

We sat around the fire telling stories, and on that night I heard from a wise old woman the very story I am about to tell you. It happened a long, long time ago. It happened, I am absolutely sure. Or perhaps it didn't. Roma had just begun their journeys through foreign lands. As a taboro moved along a long drom (road) it took them to dark, dense forests. It was frightening to be in the forest during the new moon when you couldn't see anything, and you never knew when a dangerous animal or a gang of robbers might attack you. This particular taboro made a camp on the edge of the forest with the tents set up very close together, and everyone gathered around the yag (fire), laughing, singing, chatting.

Suddenly, they heard the sound of branches crack- ing. It must be someone attracted by the fire making his way through the dark forest. Roma froze in silence and turned their heads towards the sound. Now wait, do you hear it? Ah! An old man appeared in front of them. He greeted the Roma and asked for permis- sion to warm up next to the fire. Sure! Have a seat and look at what we have here: a bowl of mushroom soup for the guest and then a strong cup of tea. First, feed the guest, then ask the questions. Who are you? Where are you coming from and where are you going?

The old man says, "Thank you for your hospitality, thank you for food and warmth. I am the Father of the Forest, Veshitko Dad. I have something to ask you. Roma travel from place to place, you go through thick forests. Are you not afraid?"

"We are very much afraid, but what are we to do but to live well with the fear?"

"Here is what I'll ask you," says the Father of the Forest. "Would you like to learn to understand the whisper of leaves, the language of trees, wild animals and birds? Would you like to feel not fear in a dark forest, but to be surrounded by protection?"

"Is there anyone who doesn't want that?" exclaimed Roma.

"I will ask something in exchange. Don't cut down my trees and don't kill wild animals and birds, do we have a deal?" Said-done. Roma agreed and as naturally as waking up from a long sleep, from that time forward they began to understand the language of trees, they communicated with wild animals and birds. They felt safe and could sense even when they could not see. I'm telling you, this is how it happened. Or not.

*H*istorically, Gypsies spent their whole lives in nature. They felt comfortable living in the forests, near lakes and rivers, walking along endless meadows, always outside, observing the seasons change, watching the Moon become full and then wane. There's an old proverb, "The one who walks a lot, knows a lot."

Romanies learned about all of the ways the Kingdom of the World communicates with us. Romanies learned this through listening to nature and experiencing how much everything is connected.

It is very important for your physical, emotional, and spiritual health to spend some time in wild places. My hope is that you are able to regularly spend time in a forest. But even going to a park or spending more time in your own backyard is better than nothing. This has to be done consistently, at least once a week.

You *must* have the time and be in places to regularly connect with the energy of the Earth, the Sky, the Sun, the Moon, the Stars, the Wind, the Trees, the Animals and the Rocks. Gypsies believe that all of these parts of nature are alive with a spirit, an essence that will help you in difficult situations.

The time you spend with nature is for connecting with the energy of different seasons. It is for receiving the healing energy from the entire Universe and giving it your love and being loved by the Kingdom in return. The natural world, the wilderness, even a park are places for inspiration, energy exercise, healing, and prayer.

If you are feeling depressed or simply out of sorts, connect with the Kingdom. If you need new ideas, go to the wilderness. If you need to mend your heart and find forgiveness for yourself and others—go to a place that has some wildness in it. The Kingdom is a place to do nothing, to just be. Smell each part of nature on your path. Lie on the grass or sit on a rock, watch the clouds move. Search for messages from the loving energy around you in the shapes of the clouds and in the behavior of the animals you meet.

Long ago Gypsies noticed that mimicking the behavior of certain animals increased health by embodying that energy. For example, if you mimic the behavior of a bear, you will feel bigger, bolder, and stronger. If you mimic the movements of a deer, you will feel agile and alert. Imitating the way a bird warms itself in the sun or devours a berry will make you feel bright and free. Because of this comfort with the natural world, Gypsies could easily train wild animals to be their partners. They recognized that each animal had a soul and was an individual, and by mimicking the behavior of an animal, they gained easier access to building communication with that animal and being at one with it.

Gypsies also believe that all other parts of nature have souls, including plants, trees, and even stones. If you haven't made friends with a stone, you've missed something special. Don't laugh until you've tried it. If you sit on a rock that feels right to you and let it give you its energy, you will feel different. Really, you will.

To begin communicating with any part of nature, you have to spend time outside. You have to get over the need to always feel comfortable, which is a terrible trap, and you have to get back in touch with the part of you that loves nature.

You are part of nature and not separate from it, and when you "get" this at a deeper level, your life will transform.

Problem: You have become accustomed to living out of touch with the cycles of nature. You spend too much time indoors and your body and soul are in danger of forgetting how to feel alive and connected to the natural world.

Solution: Get out of your comfort zone. Get out of the habit of immediately making yourself comfortable whenever you *feel* anything. Feeling is a huge part of being alive! Find a part of you that you can think of as your inner Gypsy. Don't reach for a chair to avoid sitting on the grass—sit on the grass! Sleep in a hammock or sleeping bag in your own back-yard from time to time. Let yourself feel the cold, feel the heat, feel the wind on your face, get soaked by the rain rather than maintaining a constant temperature or hiding under an umbrella. Jump into a pile of snow and bury yourself in it. Walk for hours in a forest. Learn what it feels like to be really hungry and thirsty so that food and water feel like the huge gift they really are.

Learn what it feels like to be physically exhausted from walking all day long. Build a fire and stare at the flame for a long time: not doing anything, not thinking anything, not talking, just simply looking into the fire. Gaze at the stars, notice the smells around you, follow the path of an ant to see where it leads. Mimic every movement of an animal you meet. Listen to the flow of a spring, stand under a waterfall. This will be very different from the typical hiking, camping, or backpacking experience because for the first time, you will acknowledge that everything in nature has a soul and you will feel what it's like to be in harmony with nature at the level of your soul. You will be better off not chatting with people, listening to music, or thinking about work, but making yourself so comfortable that being in nature is just like being at home. You must give yourself the gift of merging with nature in order to really feel connected, and if you begin doing that consistently, the different parts of nature will talk to you and you will feel the connection that feeds the body and soul.

Ideally you can get to beautiful and wild places often, and many people do have access to wild places. If you live near those kinds of natural resources, consider yourself deeply fortunate and take full advantage of those opportunities. If you live in an urban or suburban setting and stick to major roads, you may not be aware of how much nature is available to you. Look at a map to see how close natural places are to you and treat those places as if they are your own backyard. If you can't possibly spend time in true wilderness very often, start by searching for all of the local parks you can find. Look at a satellite photo of your city online to see where the green spaces are hiding. When I encourage someone to do this they often find that there are wonderful natural places within walking distance of where they live or work!

There is no substitution for nature and you must find a way to connect with it in order to be joyful and healthy. I'm being bossy, I know, using words like "must", but the truth can only be said very directly. During times when you cannot connect with nature on a daily basis in some way, at least *imagine* that you are connected to the natural world. Connect with the energy of the Earth and the Sky wherever you are—even in your house or in an office.

Children of the Sun

Gypsies call themselves "the children of the Sun." We say that the Sun is our father, the Moon our mother, the Earth is our grandmother, and the Sky is our grandfather. Our relationships to the cosmos are the relationships of a family. As members of the human family we are also the children and grandchildren of all of these forces.

Gypsies love the Sun, our father, and are not afraid of him. For years science has pointed people away from the sun, but that is changing. Sunscreens contain harmful chemicals. And now we understand that there are both risks to too much sun *and* conversely there are benefits from the right amount of sun. A number of recent studies demonstrate the necessity of sunlight for good health and blame a large number of deaths and certain types of cancers on vitamin D deficiency caused by *too little sunlight*!

The new recommendations are to go without sunglasses at least some of the time and to get at least 10 minutes of sun exposure every day. It is important to avoid overexposure and sunburns, but it has been shown that the benefits of moderate sun far outweigh the risks of some sun exposure.

Gypsies have always understood that the sun is a nutrient for our bodies, and now science is catching up! There is nothing new under the Sun! The new is just rediscovered ancient wisdom becoming modern scientific insight. Spend time with Father Sun and he will give you a strong heart, strong muscles, and provide wonderful energy and stamina.

Your relationship with the sun can be informed by science, common sense, and some Gypsy wisdom. The sun will help keep you in balance and is as important as everything else you take into your body. And here's another piece of Romani wisdom to consider as well—people who eat natural foods and many plants do not get sunburned to the same degree as people who eat processed food. It doesn't matter if they are light skinned and spend hours outdoors without protective clothing or sunscreen. They don't get as sunburned as easily when the nourishment they take in is full of the energy of the sun.

I was born with very pale skin. My hair was pitch black when I was born, showing my Gypsy heritage, but it has turned the warm color of sand as the years have passed. I spent my childhood in Estonia where it rains more than it shines. We have a joke in Estonia: A visitor says to an Estonian that he has heard there is no sun in Estonia. The Estonian protests, "This is not true!"

"Then why are you so pale?"

"I had to work the day the sun shone."

Because I had so little sun exposure and ate such poor quality food, any time I went to a sunny place I got severely sunburned. My skin would become red, hot, and itchy, then it would peel. Several days after the sunburn, I would still feel very uncomfortable and look absolutely hideous.

I assumed my relationship with the Sun was going to be like this for the rest of my life. But after I began eating living food, something wonderful happened: I stopped getting sunburned. I can now spend the whole day outside during the summer without wearing a hat, protective clothing, or sunscreen, and still not get sunburned. My skin gently tans and each time the sun touches my skin, I feel the tender stroke of the sun's rays that excites me. This is one of the most exhilarating feelings in the world! Be careful though: after you start eating a natural diet, it takes time for your body to remove the accumulated toxins. Depending on how much time you ate an unnatural diet, it may take several months or years for your body to be free of those toxins. But once your body has been thoroughly cleansed, you will be amazed at the way your relationship with Father Sun enhances your mood and energy and strengthens your body.

Your Mother The Moon

Gypsy wisdom refers to Mother Moon and teaches us that she is very much alive as a spiritual presence that lights the way in our own spiritual life. Science can explain how the moon and its gravitational pull effects the tides of the world's oceans, and a Gypsy will tell you about the Romani experience of the moon and how she has an impact on our emotions.

Being in communication with the moon is important to our health and to the respectful honoring of the rhythms of life. Try to start things at the new moon and complete things at the full moon. This makes use of the natural energy of the moment. Be aware that the full moon can bring about irrational behavior or high emotions, so watch yourself and be attuned so that you can counter that with rationality and a sense of calm. Or, if what wants to happen is that you go a bit wild during the full moon, give yourself permission to do that—consciously, safely, and with the proper awareness of the impact on others.

Eat in harmony with the phases of the moon. As the Moon gets fuller, so should you. Not quite as full as the Moon though. Just eat an extra apple or two. As the Moon becomes thinner, so should you. Have a juice fast for a day. Think about it this way: your body needs a variety of cycles to maintain proper balance. If you consistently eat the same amount of food every day, every week, every month, every year, you are stressing your body by making it process a great deal of food without ever stopping, slowing down, or resting. Give your body the variety of amounts of food to process and a chance to experience less. Variety and different ways of being will offer you more robust health.

Eat in accordance with the phases of the moon, and rest in accordance with your natural rhythms as well. A regular time for going to sleep and waking up is in general a good practice. But at times when you need more rest, listen to your body; it may be fighting an early illness or disease and need the boost of extra sleep. Don't push past your tiredness to be "productive" and create the deep fatigue that can host a serious illness over time.

During times when you have naturally higher levels of energy push harder, do more, and your health will benefit from the variety. You can stay up all night working or playing at times. You can spend an entire day resting in bed when you need it without any guilt about that. Variety is good for you as long as you are being responsible and do so with the intention of having good health.

All creatures with blood running through their veins are affected by the moon in ways that may be more subtle than the dramatic movement of the tides, but see what happens in your life when you dance with Mother Moon more consciously and when you surrender to the cycles of life.

*   *   *

Young children are close to the wisdom of the Kingdom and are naturally drawn to nature. They jump up at sunrise, they point excitedly at the full moon, shouting at it and saying hello. Little ones pick up leaves and chestnuts and rocks and put everything in their mouths. They stop to smell the twigs and flowers and to roll on the grass. They are fascinated by sand and dirt. They love climbing hills and touching trees. They love insects, they love animals. Think about the harm we do to them in the long run when we tell them not to touch, not to get dirty, not to engage with the natural world with passion and connection. We dampen this precious enthusiasm for the Kingdom until they forget they are a part of it.

As children grow into self-conscious teenagers, on their way to becoming limited and stiff adults, they stop engaging with the Kingdom in this wonderfully free manner. Is that what happened to you? Did you go from making mud pies to keeping clean no matter what? Not only does dirt not hurt you, it can heal you. Put your hands in it without wearing gloves and plant things. Rooting around in the dirt and its magical microbes is a gift that is close at hand but a gift we don't celebrate enough these days.

With Bare Feet

I was in a car with a friend of mine and she explained at great length the kinds of new clothes she had just bought, and where she got them, and how much she paid, and what she planned to keep and what she planned to return. I was only half listening to her and at the same time looking out the window. The sky was incredibly beautiful. It was a stunning mix of electric blues and turquoise and pure white clouds that looked as if they were illuminated from within. The view was so magnificent, so spectacular, that I interrupted my friend and said, "Look at this breathtaking gift!" My friend was baffled. She did not find the view any different than it ever was and didn't seem to think it was worth paying attention to when there were other things—like clothes—to talk about. The focus of her life was on man-made things. If she had to choose between shopping at the mall and a hike in the mountains, she would always choose the mall. With this focus, she will never be able to learn the language of nature and her life will be lived as a consumer rather than an "*experiencer*" of the richness of life.

Here's a way to let the images of nature speak to you. Talk to yourself intuitively and quickly by simply writing without thinking the answer to the question, "Who are you?" When I do this, the answers show my Gypsy point of view. "I am a river, a flower, a crystal reflecting the sun, a colorful beetle scuttling across the sand, I am moonlight, I am air." This is not an exaggeration or some romantic notion. I feel as if I am made of these things and that they are made of me.

I know that during my lifetime scientists will be able to measure the energy of our bodies and the natural world and they will see how these energies connect with much greater sophistication. I look forward to it! I'll run around and dangle the scientific proof under people's noses with delight. I want to be hooked up to whatever is invented to measure these energies while I talk to nature. I hope the contraption is given a name from the vocabulary of the Romani people. It would be fitting—we've been right about this energy stuff for a very long time you know.

$$* \quad * \quad *$$

When I need to "recharge my batteries" during the week, I go outside to plug into the Kingdom. I become like a child: I smell wild flowers, roll down the hills, and climb trees. Gypsies say the Earth gives us health and the Sun gives us joy. I encourage you to connect with the Earth and the Sun and soak up the abundant energy of life. Remember to be open to nature—don't always cover up from the sun or wear sunglasses. Don't stay comfortable and clean. Give yourself a bath in the warmth of the sun's rays. Roll in the sand. It will make such a big difference in how you feel.

I live in a city, but during the weekends I love spending time next to streams, lakes, waterfalls, and the ocean. I just watch and listen. I get wonderful ideas when I am next to sources of water in nature. Natural water is a source of great energy and information, as are the plants around us.

I planted different kinds of berries in my backyard and during the summer, I noticed a nasty weed covering all the ground between the bushes. I tried pulling it out, but it seemed to grow back overnight. So, one day, I just sat right next to it and said, "Ok, I get it. You think you should stay here. You are asserting yourself in this place. So talk to me." I listened. I could sense the plant wanted to be useful. I immediately realized that this particular weed was a stranger to me. We had never met before and I didn't know the name of the weed. I searched several Internet sites and found out that my weed was actually edible. Not only that, it turned out that it was the very delicious and nutritious purslane that had invaded my garden! Now we are friends and I'm grateful that my new friend Purslane was so insistent about making my acquaintance. I'm glad I listened.

Take any opportunity to bring parts of nature into your home: pick up and take home pine cones, leaves, acorns, chestnuts, sticks, rocks, and sea shells. Gypsies believe that these objects can be used as amulets: they protect us from evil and bring us good luck. Especially powerful are objects from nature that are shaped like an egg, an eye, a hand, a young moon, a pyramid, something that has a symmetrical shape or a very unusual shape, or that looks like an animal or a bird or has a natural hole in the middle.

I notice people looking for *perfect* sea shells on the beach and throwing down the shells they find imperfect, but I collect sea shells with a hole in the middle. There may be only one or two on the entire beach. But whenever I go to the beach, I ask that these shells find me. I may walk for ten minutes without looking down and then stop, look down and see a little shell. I pick it up, wash it in the water and find out that it has a hole in the middle! It is as if I am magnetized to them or they are magnetized to me. They bring me good luck, these *imperfect* and less valuable shells. I go looking for good luck and appreciate it when I hold it in my hand.

Remember the song? "There's a crack, a crack in everything. That's how the light gets in." Value is in the eye of the beholder, and the imperfect, broken, inexpensive, or free can have the most value of all. I am delighted by my shells with holes. What can you invite into your life to celebrate its imperfection, impermanence, and the joy and luck of small things?

*   *   *

If you will remember just one thing from this book, let it be this. Remember to walk barefoot outside as often as you can. Roma say, "Who walks in tight boots has blisters, who walks barefoot has none." The meaning of this is not just about the difference between walking barefoot or in boots. It means that being constrained and booted is not as good for the soul as feeling connected to the Earth.

Walking barefoot is a way of taking your place in the Kingdom. Do you feel more comfortable being barefoot in your own house than you would in other situations? Do you enjoy being barefoot at home? There's a reason for that. You are *home*, you are *comfortable*, it is your *special place*! You take your shoes off to signify this without realizing that is what you are doing. The wisdom of your body is telling you something and you unconsciously act in response. But now that you know this, you can be more conscious about it.

You need to feel that all of nature is your *home* in order to be truly whole. The healing energy of the Earth is for you. The Kingdom will teach you everything you need to know in order to be healthy and happy—if you touch it with your bare feet and listen. Walk barefoot on the ground, on the grass, on the sand, on the rocks, and in the streams. Run barefoot in the snow.

When I was a child, my mother told me to walk barefoot as much as possible. She was repeating what her mother, her grandmother, and her great-grandmother had told her. In Russian and Gypsy villages, kids run barefoot all summer long. When I spent the summer months in the camp, I would only walk barefoot. These were the happiest of days because I was deeply connected to nature.

If you visit sacred lands, take off your shoes and your socks. Many traditions insist that you remove your shoes before entering sacred spaces. It is so that you can really connect with those places. See! I told you! Walk barefoot to connect with holy energy any chance you get and you will become very peaceful and happy. At the same time, you will feel a surge of energy. The energy will feel as if it "bubbles up" or "rises" inside of you through the soles of your bare feet. At some point, it will rise to the top of your head and you will have a creative idea that will seem to come from nowhere, but in fact came from the Earth under your feet.

When you can't take off your shoes, use your hands. Touch the grass, touch the leaves, hug the trees (you may want to ask their permission first). Feel the heaviness of stones in your hands. To feel an even deeper connection with nature, sing with the birds, talk to the plants, stretch as if you are trying to touch the sky.

Beauty produces spontaneous feelings of connection with the entire Universe and can be found all around you. People will save up their money and travel thousands of miles to visit lovely places, but forget to appreciate what is close at hand. Love and send thanks to the flowering bush on your block. Have a close relationship with the birds in your neighborhood. Gypsy wisdom tells us that everything has a spirit. Love and appreciate those spirits and let those spirits love you.

Problem: You work all day in an office that does not have windows, or your home doesn't have a strong connection to nature.

Solution: Transform the places you spend time in by inviting nature in with plants, pictures of nature, fountains, bowls of sand, pine cones, acorns, chestnuts, sticks, rocks, and sea shells. Tend to bird feeders and the plants that naturally attract them. If there are no sounds of nature around you, at least play recordings of the sounds of birds, the sea, and the wind in the places in which you live and work. Once in a while, stop what you are doing and direct your attention to the big tree next to your office. Even if you can't see it from your office window, it's there, and you are connected to it and its healing energy. Just take a few seconds to acknowledge and thank that tree and visit it when you eat your lunch—outside.

Problem: You experience high stress and a feeling of being burned out, but you only have a few minutes to recuperate.

Solution: Go outside, take off your shoes and socks and walk barefoot on grass, let the wind mess up your hair, listen to the birds. Don't think about anything; just be in complete harmony with nature for a few minutes. This is the best way to transform high stress into bliss.

Today I am sitting in my office looking outside the window. The window is the gate between two worlds: my office is filled with problems, questions, and stress, and the natural world is there to fill me with quiet contemplation, beauty and bliss.

I close my eyes and in my imagination I sneak out as if I have stepped through the gate and journeyed into nature. I stay there for a while. I enjoy walking on air. I smile and open my eyes. Nothing changed inside my office, but for those few minutes everything changed inside of me. I am calm and strong. And problems? Bring them on!

*   *   *

It all starts with the most powerful healer—Nature herself. Nature gives us everything we are made of and everything we make. We breathe her, drink her, bask in her light and beauty, connect with her stars, and learn from her animals, plants, and even the stones of the Earth. There is wisdom in the trees, power in the mountains, and magic in the moon. We get in trouble and we get sick when we replace Nature with the artificial world, and we thrive when we make the choice to connect with the Kingdom.

Imagine The Wild

Before you start this game, open the windows and air everything out for at least thirty minutes. Let the stagnant energy escape from the room and invite new energy in. If it's hot air outside, let it be hot. If it's cold air, let it be cold. If you take my advice you are going to get more comfortable with being uncomfortable and being with nature as it is. Sit looking out the window (if you have a beautiful view) or looking at a picture of nature if you do not. Turn on a CD with the sounds of nature—songs of birds or waves crashing. Or listen to a small fountain. Close your eyes.

Imagine the most magnificent place in nature that you have ever seen yourself in person, or have seen in a film or a book or on the Internet. It can be on top of a mountain, on a beach, in a forest. If it is the beach, imagine what it feels like to sit on the sand, scoop some sand into your hands, let it warm your palms, let it sift through your fingers. Run into the water, swim underwater. Anything is possible here because you are imagining, so let your imagination run wild—literally. Talk to the fish, ride a dolphin. Your brain is capable of richly imagining a wilderness experience and a connection to nature—so make good use of it and go deeply into this realm.

Now, imagine that you are flying. Imagining that you are flying will help anyone to feel more freedom and will put you in a good mood right away. Gypsies tell stories about how they were once birds. Now in the twenty-first century you can find footage on the Internet of people flying in wing suits at over one hundred miles per hour. This may be for people who are young, strong, and dangerously risk-taking, but for a reasonable amount of money you can actually fly very safely in a wind tunnel to experience a little taste of the feeling. For the rest of your life you can recreate it in your body whenever you want. What a wonderful combination of science and magic!

Imagining yourself as a bird is very healing. Stretch your arms out. Take a deep breath. Smile! Imagine looking at your home from a bird's eye view. What does your roof look like? Now fly anywhere you wish, look at the world from above, bask in the Sun's rays, fly high through the clouds.

We are unusual birds now because we are Romanies, so you can take a break from flying and jump through a cloud, wash your face with snow newly formed and falling as you fly, imagine it dissolving in your mouth. There are no rules and you can break the laws of nature and invent new ones if you wish. Do what makes you happy. When you are ready to land, open your eyes and stretch. You've just improved your physical, emotional, and even spiritual health by playing with nature, even if you haven't had access to the real thing on this particular day. Magic can always come from inside you.

Animals Will Tell You

If you would like to learn how the Universe communicates with you through nature, notice what kinds of animals show up in your life. Is there a pattern to the kind of birds that fly directly over your head? Are they the same kinds of birds? Does their appearance seem to punctuate something in your life? Maybe someone gave you a calendar with dogs. Your friend asked you to take care of her dog while she is out of town. A pair of doves are nesting outside your window and softly calling. You keep noticing art with a tiger in it, or your eye is being drawn to images of rabbits, and so on. Think about the behavior and spirit of that animal that is showing up in your personal world. For example, if you "accidently" sit on an anthill, don't see that as a random event and ask yourself, "Am I feeling too isolated and passive and could use some brisk activity with lots of other people around to heal my body and soul?" Perhaps an encounter with an anthill will help you understand that you are working too hard and that you never have time just for yourself. Engage in an internal conversation based on what you observe and experience in nature— speak to it and let it speak to you in symbols.

When I was writing this book, I reached a point where I got very stuck didn't have any ideas, and my enthusiasm was drained. Even my magical notebook did not help (I have a notebook that I have created that "makes" me write). I just could not write any more for some reason and I couldn't understand it. The next day I went to work as usual, and the day was no different from my other days at work. But in the afternoon, a co-worker entered my office, beaming. She was excited about a goose that had laid her eggs right next to the entrance of a nearby building, a short walk from my office. I didn't even think about this incident being a possible sign that I could read to benefit my life. But my co-worker was so animated and she would not stop talking about the geese. The weather was beautiful and I decided to take a look at them as an excuse to take a walk.

We watched the mother goose sitting on her eggs. She was full of nurturing energy. She was warming up the life beneath her. We read some facts about geese taped to the glass door by someone who wanted to help protect them and then we went back to work.

I forgot about the mother goose until the next morning when I grabbed a plate for breakfast and noticed an illustration of the bird in the corner of my plate. I was surprised. I had washed this plate hundreds of times and never even noticed the goose! There are so many other designs on this beautiful Gypsy plate and I had never examined it closely. I began thinking about this little discovery when I remembered the goose outside. The Kingdom was whispering wisdom and I had almost ignored it. Birds often appear to those who need to feel more connected to their souls and their largest potential. I sat down to write in my magic notebook about the desires of my soul and to explore what was really possible in my life.

I listened to this wisdom of animals and the symbols they whispered. I stopped everything and connected with the birds, and I was filled with new energy, my mind as full of ideas as there are feathers on a goose. When you feel stuck, take this advice—spend time with birds, mimic their flight, imagine yourself flying high into the sky and returning from that higher altitude with great ideas.

Wisdom in The Trees

If there are no animals showing up in your life, start paying attention to the trees around you. Gypsies have a very special relationship with trees. We see trees as alive, thinking, and emotional beings. We have lived in trees, slept in them, hidden high in their branches to be safe from harm. We know that a tree can laugh and that it can cry. It can make jokes, take away pain, and share wisdom. It will give you food, provide cool shade in the unrelenting heat, and provide fire to sustain you. Trees literally give us the breath of life—oxygen. Gypsies knew that trees could breathe and that they shared their special energy with us long before science did because we knew trees as our close friends.

Trees have been the main source of fire for thousands of ages, but for Gypsies, they are also a source of the "spiritual fire" of our lives. They give us support and they teach us to use unspoken communication.

If you want a better life, plant trees, care for them, talk to them. Trees, like mountains, are the link between the Upper, Middle and Lower Spiritual Worlds. Their roots are deep in the Earth, their trunks are above the ground, and their branches touch the sky. Become friends with a particular tree. Find a big, wise, old tree somewhere and invite it to be your special tree. Use your intuition to select the tree and ask for permission to get acquainted. If you become friends, the tree will take your wishes to the Lower and Upper Worlds and will help make sure your wishes come true. Trees existed on Earth long before people appeared, and some very special trees have even more power than animals.

My very first childhood memory is of pine trees so tall that I couldn't see the tops of the trees when I craned my head up to the sky. I had a special relationship with one particular tree and I would approach it with respect and gently touch it. My hand would get sticky from pine resin and it would remain on my palms for hours, scenting everything I touched. Once in a while I would raise my hand to my nose to inhale the sharp smell. The scent of pine resin is powerfully cleansing and I inhale it every chance I get. I also collect pine cones and bring them home, so that I can welcome the spirit of a pine tree into my life indoors. Essential oils that come from trees possess an extraordinary ability to awaken psychic powers. At the end of the book, I will teach you how to access them.

I know people who are similarly fed by the desert. That environment doesn't speak to me personally in the same way as a dense forest does, but you'll know what is right for you because nature will meet you in the right resonance. Enjoy your experience of the Kingdom with your whole heart and in your own way. I'm grateful for the role trees have played in this book—it was written next to some of my favorite trees, and as one of the ways it's delivered to readers, it is printed on trees as well. I will continue to plant trees to help keep everything in balance and to express my gratitude for the writing and sharing of this book.

In what ways does nature provide for you in your life? Take a moment and look at the objects around you—the wool rug, the plant, the stone, the iron bar that provides support, the gold that glints on your finger. How does nature provide for you in your work and in your life at home? What can you do to feel that connection more keenly?

Problem: You feel disconnected from nature.
Solution: To connect with the Kingdom of the World, pretend you are a tree, an animal, a stone, or a flower. What kind of spirit would you have? How would you move or stay rooted? What feelings or thoughts would you have? Go for a walk every day, even

if it is only a short one. Notice the dew on the leaves. Search for rainbows when it rains. Watch the clouds move. Admire them. Without clouds, there is no rain, there is no life. Look at the bees. Thank them for their work when they cross your path. Without bees, there is no pollination; there is no life. Bees are disappearing. Talk to them about this. The more you observe and interact with nature, the more you'll understand the connectedness of all the elements of the world, and the more nature will talk to you and heal you.

Problem: Your daily patterns are too fixed and you don't feel the magic of your days and nights. You have lost touch with sunrises and sunsets and you look more at the face of the clock than the face of the moon. You are not connected to the energy and essence of the day or night.

Solution: Greet the sun in the morning and say good night to the sun in the evening. If you are usually a night owl, try going to bed with the sun and waking before dawn. This will help you appreciate your connection to time and the turning of day to night and night to day. Sunrise and sunset are times of powerful energy, but unfortunately in the modern world we are often busiest and most distracted during those magical times of the day. Tuning into the beginning and ending of days will help you connect with more of the life force you need to be healthy and joyful.

Watch the phases of the moon. They are important. Our bodies are mostly water, and the tides and the water of the world are connected to the moon. Listen to the wisdom of your body and how it connects with the larger Universe and our small place in it—this beautiful planet brimming with life.

$\mathcal{T}hree$

KISSING THE PEACH

Your Future In What You Eat

$\mathcal{H}$istorically, Gypsies have lived in situations where it has been difficult to store food. We say, "A Rom is not a squirrel, he'll survive without storing food." For several centuries, there was only one meal a day—dinner. It would always be freshly made with lots of greens (sorrel being the favorite).

As you know, food can be a very powerful medicine or a poison. Food can heal and food can kill. Food has enormous power. Depending on what's on your plate, how much food there is, and how it got there, food can nourish your body and spirit or destroy them. We have known this forever, and now science is finally saying the same thing. Whatever you eat becomes your future.

If you eat food with low energy (food out of a can or a box), you will not feel the hunger in your body, but your body will be starving for nutrition and you will be unwell.

If you eat food with high energy (uncooked, fresh, close to the source of the Earth that made it), you will leave the table without feeling stuffed and your body will be well nourished and full of energy. Eat food that is as close as possible to the way nature created it and you will have clarity of mind and a powerful body.

Pay attention for the next few days to exactly what you eat and think about the reality that what you eat will very literally become who you are:

- Where did the food you are about to eat come from?
- Can you point to a place on the map where it was grown? The farther from your home, the less energy it will have for you.
- Do you personally know the people who grew your food? Are they kind, caring people? Their energy will enter your body along with the food.
- Was this food stored for months (or even years!) on a shelf or in a freezer? The longer it takes from the time food was picked to the time it reaches your plate, the less life force the food will have.
- If someone prepared it in a commercial kitchen or in a home, was it made with care and intention?

Let's play a game called, "Is it living or dead?" I will only let you do this if you approach this game with love and good humor. If you're going to feel guilty or ashamed about what you discover, you aren't allowed to do it. I'm not kidding. Don't mess with me, I'm a Gypsy. There is nothing about this exploration that should end up making you feel worse about yourself and your life. My intention is only to bless you.

We're going to look at your food closely to see how much of what you eat is really good for you. We're going to see if your health and your ability to live joyfully are supported by what you take into your body.

The Game: Go to your pantry, cupboards, refrigerator, and freezer, open everything up, and look carefully at what you eat. Think about the food you eat when you are out at a restaurant or going through a drive through window. What are your snacks? Be honest about what you see. What do you eat most often? What sits uneaten? When you eat out, what do you choose? Put all of this food on a table in your imagination and assess it honestly. Whatever you see is the picture of your future health. Will your body be processed, pickled, canned, dried out, boxed up, frozen? Or will it be vibrant, beautiful, colorful, full of life and juice, and be really and truly *fresh*?

What You Do Next: If you don't see enough fresh food to fuel a good life, start your grocery shopping in the produce section first to fill up your basket with colorful and vibrant living things that are truly good for you as your top priority.

Tempt yourself into better habits by leaving a beautiful cook book with photos of beautifully prepared fresh food open on the kitchen counter, or your dining room table. Place the open book where you and your family will be inspired to use it.

Find your local farmer's market and make walking there to buy local produce a habit.

Display fruit that is ripening in beautiful bowls in your home where you'll see it and want to eat it before you unconsciously reach for less nutritious options.

Arrange the shelves of your refrigerator so that fresh food is displayed like a treasure in beautiful colored bowls and plates. No plastic or opaque containers please, use only beautiful glass that shows off your good food and seduces your pallet when you see it. The investment in good things to display and care for your food is the smartest money you can spend. You are creating your future body. Love it!

* * *

My daughter is a teenager and easily embarrassed by me these days, but I like to explore the produce section and let myself be drawn to unfamiliar fruits, vegetables, and herbs. "What's that and how can I use it?" I ask the green grocer, who is usually delighted to be able to talk about what is offered. My daughter thinks that I am making a fool of myself when I ask tons of questions. But she passionately consumes *whatever it is* once I figure out how to fix it well.

Food that has the highest spiritual energy and the most nutrition is food you grow yourself, pick yourself, and eat right away. It still carries magical, life-giving energy that will move right into your body and will give you great health.

The next best food is grown by people you know and trust. And then everything moves down the list of what is desirable to the very worst food which is made without any care and with exploited labor and bad practices that harm the environment. Not only is this food without a soul, but it can even carry negative energy that is harmful to you as well.

I recommend that you eat everything with the question, "What future am I eating?" Take a moment to consider what kind of energy you are taking into your body. Fruit and greens have the energy of the Sun: eat them when you don't have enough energy and when you are tired or sick. Vegetables have the energy of the Earth: eat them when you need to be grounded or have too much energy or feel distracted and restless. Nuts have the energy of life locked inside of them. To release it, soak them in spring water overnight, then discard the water and rinse the nuts well. Wild food has the magical energy of intuition. Eat it if you need to increase your insight. High quality essential oils added to a meal will turn it into medicine healing your body. Only use essential oils I recommend at the end of the book. Avoid adding essential oils sold in regular stores that may not be safe. I hope this is connecting with you on several levels because if you make these simple changes, they will transform your health and your life.

The Food of Love

Gypsy wisdom has it that there is dead food that will sap your energy and make you sick and living food that will give you energy and good health. In the modern world, we know that conventional food is dead food. It lacks vitamins and minerals and is loaded with chemicals, hormones, and antibiotics. If we could travel back in time to the nomadic way of living with the Roma, we would see that they ate what was available to them during the season of the year and in that particular place. They ate wild plants, but they had made a deal with Veshitko Dad that they would not eat wild animals because those animals were sacred. Roma would only eat domesticated animals. They also enjoyed foods that are no longer common. Gypsies collected and drank birch juice by tapping the birch tree. During colder months they ate wild mushrooms.

Eating simply is a pleasure that will put you in touch with the Kingdom. Here's a very simple Romani recipe.

Shred a crisp cabbage and place it in a beautiful bowl. Aesthetics matter in making and eating food properly, so a beautiful bowl is part of this recipe. If you don't have one—go get one, or ask someone you know who has many beautiful bowls and who cooks with love if you can have one of theirs because it will carry that history of good energy with it. We don't always have to go out to buy something new when something that is old has wonderful energy in it. Music and conversation are also good ingredients to add to food. So now that you are working with beautiful things and listening to music and talking to people you love--here's the rest of the recipe. Squeeze the juice out of the cabbage with your hands and add some shredded carrots and beets and any fresh herbs you have on hand—dill, cilantro, parsley, mint. Add a dash of apple cider vinegar and perhaps a little garlic and some fresh ginger and a bit of olive oil and a pinch of black pepper and sea salt or salt from high in the Himalayan Mountains. Mix well and let the salad sit on the counter for an hour to marinate the flavors and let them mix together. This is a meal that will make you happy and healthy and feed your spirit and the spirit of others who eat it with you.

Cooking food destroys much of the energy and nutrition in the food, so if you must, cook things as lightly as possible. Trust nature; nature is the best chef. When food is alive, you can talk to your food, ask it to heal you, and observe amazing changes happening in your body.

From a traditional Gypsy perspective, the relationship many Americans have with food seems odd. On the one hand there is the extreme of eating large quantities of food that isn't really feeding the body because it has no nutrients and it doesn't really taste good anyways. People are eating this bad food with absolutely no sense of enjoyment. They stuff their faces without any joy. There is nothing nutritious about that experience for the body or soul. A big nasty meal at a fast food restaurant eaten quickly is not a celebration of life that leaves you feeling great, it is a habit that will literally kill you.

Then there is the problem of taking too much pleasure in eating food that is too full of fat, sugar, salt, and flavor additives designed by food companies to overwhelm the pallet and to literally be addictive to your brain. This is a huge part of the food industry—the behind-the-scenes manipulation of flavors to get you hooked on something that doesn't come from nature and that is designed to create more desire for that particular amped-up artificial flavor that only that food created by that company can provide.

The modern diet tends to focus on a false sort of feeling good by loading up with foods that are mistaken as being there for "comfort" but in reality leave you uncomfortable, tired, and unhealthy.

Gypsy wisdom recommends the deeper pleasure that comes from eating really delicious food that is also really good for you in the company of people you really love. That is a good life, good health, and good nutrition!

To get the most energy from your food, you have to be happy while eating. That's why the dining atmosphere and food presentation are so important. Traditional Romani meals are served with all the family present and no distractions from enjoying each other—just talking (no texting) and laughing and eating together.

Don't let your family eat in front of the television or computer or with their cell phones in their hands. Sit together and concentrate on the good feeling you have for each other and your appreciation for the food you eat and your life will be full of joy.

Animals and kids play with their food—and even though my teenage daughter is preoccupied with acting cool these days, she actually kisses a perfect peach before she eats it because she is so overwhelmed with joy. I was inspired to write a song for her that I now play on my guitar and share with audiences and with my taboro:

Life is a peach
Juicy delicious
Life is a storm
Cleansing and powerful
Life is a dream
Vivid and colorful
Come to the feast
Dance in the storm
Follow your dream
Life is a peach!

We can learn a great deal from someone who is close to nature and has enthusiasm for life. One of my favorite places to eat is a café that serves fresh, live, organic raw food and every dish includes *love* right there in the ingredient list printed on the menu. Look for these kinds of places, family run special places where people actually care about what they serve you. There are food resources that are right under your nose that will offer you love and nutrition. There are places of refuge and regeneration in places that will surprise you. Don't look for the usual. Seek the unusual. Don't sleep your way into buying the recognized brand. Find the little treasures in your neighborhood and then share them with your taboro.

Do Not Eat Your Pain

Remember this as you reach for your food. Ask your body and your soul what your state of mind is and how your emotions feel to you. Don't eat when you are stressed or angry. The energy of the food and your energy will not match and it will create havoc inside your body. Eat only when you are physically hungry. A lot of people eat when they are "emotionally hungry" or when they are bored without realizing that this is what they are doing and so they are never satisfied and never happy. Their bodies will naturally carry extra weight because of the "weightiness" of their concerns while eating it.

Start treating yourself with more love and care. Pay careful attention to your emotional needs. Are you frightened, hurt, lonely, sad? Don't eat when you feel activated in these ways. Drink a cup of water and then go *do* something interesting instead! Process those emotions by talking to people you love and who you know will feed you emotional support. Write how you feel. Take ownership for the *hunger* you feel. Do you want to be creative? Are you hungry for affection? Are you hungry for more meaning in your life? Name your hunger and act on it with passion because this hunger will lead you to a better life, romantic partner, a job with a sense of calling. Hunger will teach you!

Have you noticed that people who are in love don't think about food? And those who are depressed tend to eat more? When food is sought out wrongly to provide happiness, you don't see joy in anything else. You resign yourself to the thought that life will not bring you magic. In that situation, food will not nourish you but will numb you and bury you in excess weight rather than setting you free to live your life with energy and power in a body that is just the right size for you. If you eat well, you'll notice the world around you. You will look deeply into another person's eyes. You will feel your own heart.

The wrong food will make you too full and lethargic and always tired, and you still won't be able to sleep well. Eating when you are not hungry, overeating, and eating food with low energy will make you sick now and later on. I also see a common problem with my clients that is a disturbing pattern common in our culture. Many people have a lazy habit of watching television at night and eating instead of bringing their healthy hunger and energy to their partner in the bedroom. When the sun sets it's time to share intimacy, not more calories. Sooner or later a body stuffed with bad food becomes a weak body that doesn't have the energy to connect with others.

Loving Moderation

If you are not always busy digesting food, you will feel more attentive, more present, more attuned to others and your surroundings. You will be so alert and you will have so much energy that you will not be able to sit still. It's amazing how much energy is spent on the task of digesting heavy food in large quantities, and until you experience the great freedom of eating less but much better quality food, you may not know it down to your cells. I promise you, the difference is extraordinary! But you'll only know for sure if you try it.

Yes, there are times when there should be a ton of food on the table. These are special and rare occasions that are times to celebrate, to share, and to acknowledge life's bounty. Eating until you are very full has its place during special holidays and big occasions. This is a rare pleasure. Don't make it an everyday habit or you will falsely "celebrate" your body into illness.

In my family, the biggest celebration of life is going skiing, hiking, swimming, or dancing. I've never, not once, been to an American party where people eat just the right amount and then get up and dance and dance. Yet that's how most Russian and Gypsy gatherings are conducted. Imagine a Thanksgiving where your family eats some really good quality food and then someone turns on the music, and you all (including grandparents and great-grandparents) get up and dance! Try it!

Roma say, "If you eat a lot, you will not dance well," and we also say, "Happiness is not in drinking and eating, but in the singing and the dancing."

* * *

There are so many reasons not to overeat—it's not good for the planet because it uses up too many resources and it's not good for

individual people because it shortens their lives. It's not good for
couples because it saps their energy for each other. It's not good for
families because it ruins their collective health and instills bad habits
in the next generations. We say, "Rom has mostly tendons and skin
and is thin, yet he's healthy and strong and happy."

Many years have passed and much water has flowed
under many bridges since the time this story happened. There was a Romani family who lived poorly. Often, there were not even bread crumbs for the
children. Everyone was hungry, and always asking a
Romny (Gypsy woman) for food. So the Romny went
into the forest and asked the Father of the Forest,
"Veshitko Dad, help me, poor dzhuvly (woman): my
children are crying, asking for food. Where am I to
find it?" Suddenly, there appeared the Father of the
Forest and he said, "I see you are a good, kind woman.
I will help you. I will teach you how to find nourishing
wild food and how to avoid poisonous food. Simply
come here and say, "Food, appear!" At this very moment, everything that is not safe to eat will disappear.
When you are done gathering food, say, "Thank you!"
and everything will go back to its place. Only take as
much as you can carry in your apron, enough to feed
your family for one day." He said this and vanished.

So the Romny looked around and whispered, "Food, appear," and right away she saw a sea of plants, flowers, berries, and mushrooms. She filled her apron and said, "Thank you!" and everything went back to its place. From that time, this Romani family always had just the right amount of food.

Living and Dead Water

When I was a child, my mother took me to a small town on the shore of the Black Sea. We didn't have a place to stay, so we went from house to house asking for a room to rent, but none were available. It was a popular town right on the beach and it attracted many tourists.

It was getting darker with each minute. We had spent the whole day searching and still had no place to stay. Finally, exhausted, we knocked on the door of a beautiful white house right next to a white rock mountain. I was mesmerized by this mountain. Somehow I knew that I had just discovered something that would have important meaning in my life.

My mother knocked on the door. A woman appeared and told us that there were no rooms available. Then she looked at me. I was still under the spell of the amazing mountain. The woman kept looking into my eyes. Suddenly, she turned to my mom and said: "I will let you stay in my room. Your daughter has the most unusual eyes I've ever seen."

We had a wonderful vacation. I climbed on the rocks of the white mountain and spent hours just sitting on them and resting my hands on their surface. I talked to them and they talked to me.

The sea was warm and the beaches had pebbles that created the most unusual sound when they rolled over each other in the surf. It was paradise.

I wanted to return soon, but it wasn't until twenty-five years later that I got a chance to come back, and it happened as if by magic. I knew at some point in my life I would have to find a way to return to that special place because it is very important to fulfill your childhood dream. Did you know this? It is a magical idea and needs to be acted upon, even if you don't understand it. Someone very wise once said, "Truly I tell you, unless you change and become like little children, you will never enter the kingdom of heaven."

Take a moment and remember your childhood dreams. What can you do to act upon them in some way? There are deep, spiritual, and practical reasons for your dreams, and you will only decode the secret once you connect your life as an adult to your life as a child.

When I returned to one of the most sacred places of my childhood, I was guided there. I had been staying in a healing center, and one of the staff members recommended a particular massage therapist who unfortunately didn't have any slots left. I felt intuitively that I needed to have a massage from *her*. From the early morning until late at night her schedule was full. But I wouldn't leave. Just like when I was a kid asking for what my soul needed, I stood there looking into her eyes because I knew something important wanted to happen. She was silent for a moment and then she said "All right, come in today after everyone's gone and I'll stay later."

I already knew that a good massage can create a miracle, but this was a new experience for me. She used two methods: one that warms up the skin and the other that warms up the muscles. Together, they created a feeling of immense internal heat, similar to the feeling you'd get in a sauna. But there were two magical reasons for me needing to meet this massage therapist. The first was that she taught me about living water.

Living water? I was intrigued because this idea connected with things I had heard about Gypsy wisdom in my childhood. I pulled a bottle of spring water from my backpack and asked her if it was alive. She laughed. No, no, of course it wasn't. Everything that was bottled is no longer alive. And of course the water from a tap is not alive either, because it is chemically treated. If you drink directly from a clean spring, you drink water that has the live energy of the Earth, the rocks, the trees around it, the Sun, the Moon and the Stars. If you drink water from a freshly opened young coconut or freshly made juice, it is *water* that is wonderfully alive. Bottled spring water, tap water, distilled water, boiled water, and any other liquid that is bottled or canned is dead. It no longer has life-giving energy.

Gypsy wisdom teaches us that the most magical water, the best water, hides from the sun. It's found in dark, cool places and comes from the depths of the Earth. Once you become accustomed to living water, you can instantly tell the difference. And here is a secret. It is relatively easy to find springs of living water, even in a large city. There are maps on the internet to show you where to find natural springs, and it is understood that people will help themselves to this wonderful water.

Begin with what you have and work your way up with every chance you have to make a choice. If you must drink bottled water, make sure that the quality of the bottled water is better than tap water. If you have to drink tap water, make sure to filter it because it contains chemicals and drug residue. And there are a few little tricks to bring water back to life. In the old days a Gypsy would put a piece of pure silver in the water. You might try putting all the water you drink, even filtered water, through an inexpensive wine aerator that creates a vortex of energy and fills the water with oxygen as a way of drinking water that is one step closer to living water every day. It's also a good idea to put a few drops of fresh lemon juice and to vigorously stir the water before you drink it to give it life again. The easiest way to add life to water is to add high quality essential oils. Use the ones I recommend at the end of the book and never add essential oils to water in plastic containers. Don't add essential oils sold in regular stores to your water. They may not be safe. And if you want some bigger magic with your water, place spring or filtered water in a clear glass container with a tight lid in the bright moonlight, but remember to put it in the dark and cold refrigerator in the morning before the sun takes the life back out of it.

You will be amazed at the amount of energy you will have when you drink living water. It will transform your body. I was grateful to the massage therapist for offering this life changing advice, and I made another appointment with her a few days after our first one. When I arrived, she was still busy with a previous client. I sat down on a comfortable couch in the waiting room and thumbed through the newspapers and magazines on the table. Suddenly, I stopped as if I had been jolted with electricity. There was a photograph of "my" magical mountain, the place from my childhood that I had been so desperate to return to. The town right next to Alupka was called Simeiz. The translation of this word from Greek means "Signs." The author took pictures of several mountains surrounding Simeiz. One of them looked like a cat and was named, well, the Cat Mountain. Several mountains looked like pyramids and were known to collect and distribute spiritual energy; the Black Sea served as a mirror. I intuitively knew these mountains were special when I was a kid. Now I knew why.

I kept reading. I found out that there are ninety-five dolmens on the Cat Mountain. Dolmens are made from megaliths, or huge stones (think of Stonehenge). Some of them are ten thousand years old. In Romani tradition, dolmens are gates to the Otherworld (unseen spiritual world). I had followed my intuition and would now be able to fulfill a childhood wish. She had opened the door to my childhood dream and had also given me the gift of living water. Her last client left. It was my turn! The magic of life is often found in these unexpected connections.

Sit closer to me. I will tell you a story. This story is whispered, very quietly. Pay attention. This is a story about the dead and living water.

There once was a king. He was rich beyond measure. He owned vast tracts of land, several castles, many horses, and had chests full of gold and precious stones. Yet he was very unhappy: he was old, sick, and blind. To entertain himself, he invited a Gypsy choir to sing for him. The Roma came and they sang and sang. One song touched the king's heart the most. "What is this song about?" asked the king. One Gypsy volunteered to translate. "This song is about live and dead water. Living water heals and brings back the ability to see. Dead water takes away strength and makes you sick and weak. Far-far away, high in the mountains, there are two sources of water: one with dead water and one with living water. One who finds water that is full of the life of the Kingdom will never die."

The king got excited, "Tell me, Gypsy, is it true? Does the live water exist?" "Who knows? Maybe it's true," said the Gypsy.

The king sent his servants to announce to the entire kingdom: One who finds live water will get his kingdom and everything in it. So the old and the young began searching for the live water. They went deep into thick forests, they climbed high mountains, avoiding only one the highest. Rumor had it that there lived a dragon who ate anyone passing by.

But one Gypsy did not go into the forests and did not climb the mountains. He was sleeping calmly under a tree. During his sleep he had a strange dream: In it he climbed the highest mountain and met the dragon. The dragon flew toward him, fire erupting from its mouth. The Gypsy saw himself using a sharp sword to kill the dragon. Was it a dream or a vision?

The Gypsy woke up, not knowing what to make of this. He thought about it and finally decided to climb the tallest mountain. He climbed for two days. Close to the top of the mountain, he saw a lake. The water was so calm it looked like a mirror. Suddenly, he saw a reflection of the dragon in the lake. The dragon flew at him, fire erupting from its mouth, burning his hands and face. This is when the Gypsy realized that he did not have a sword. Desperate, he took off one of his boots, filled it with water from the lake and poured the water on the dragon's head. The dragon fell to the ground and died. "This is the dead water," gasped the Gypsy. He walked around the lake and saw a spring of water coming from deep inside the mountain. The water ran very fast as if it was dancing, and it was very cold and came from a place deep in the Earth.

The Gypsy washed his hands and his face with the water, and his painful burns healed. He filled his flask with the living water and delivered it to the king. The king drank the water and used it to wash his eyes. He could see better and felt as if he had the energy of a young man. As he promised, the king gave his kingdom to the Gypsy and his taboro. Now that he had no possessions to guard and worry about, the king rode off on a great horse to travel to see the world and to tell the story of the living water. The king told this story to someone who told it to me.

Dead and living water really do exist, and understanding the difference will improve the quality of your life. The difference between the Gypsy folk tale and the life we are living in the Middle World is that dead water will not kill you right away, but it will make you sick over time. And living water will not make you immortal, but it will give you amazing health, energy, and a longer life.

Problem: Frequent colds, aches and pains.

Solution: Start adding as much live water and live food to your diet as you can. Make fresh juices (combine four big stalks of celery, half a lemon, half an inch of ginger, a big bunch of dark leafy greens, one apple, one carrot, one small peeled beet) and visit a juice bar regularly. Eat lots of fresh fruit. Eat a big salad before each meal. Russians say, "Sweet kills; bitter heals." Reduce sweets and add bitter greens (dandelion, nettles, radish tops) and garlic.

Problem: You don't have money to buy fancy organic produce. You don't have a place to grow much yourself. It seems daunting to change your diet.

Solution: Have fun with this challenge and get in touch with your inner Gypsy. Buy what is in season and buy when your favorite fruits and vegetables are on sale. Approach the manager of a health food store and ask to pick up produce that they intend to throw away at the end of the day. You will be surprised to find out that perfectly fine food is being thrown out and that when you ask for it they will let you have it. Carrot tops, radish tops, beet tops, and turnip tops can all be juiced with celery and lemon for a delicious and nutritious drink. Visit your local farmers market at the end of the day and you can get a big discount and even free food! Grow wonderful sprouts inside a jar for only a few cents. Grow your own food and herbs in little pots if you only have a little space. Go foraging: nature is abundant with free food (attend a class to learn what's edible and what's not). Join a food co-op and buy in bulk. Join a CSA (community supported agriculture) program and volunteer in exchange for fruits and vegetables. Ask your co-workers or neighbors to let you make good use of the extra fruit and vegetables from their gardens: they often can't eat it all and end up throwing a lot away and feeling guilty about it. They will love giving it to you. You see how fun resource-fulness can be?

The Mushroom Kingdom

For hundreds of years Gypsies survived on the most nutritious food—wild food. Foraging was a big part of a woman's day. She would bring home wild fruits and berries, edible weeds, greens and flowers, wild roots and herbs, grasses and nuts, even young pine needles and tree and bush leaves. But the most important and filling wild foods were mushrooms.

I was four years old when my grandfather first took me to a forest to gather mushrooms. I will never forget it. The weather was chilly and wet; we wore high rain boots, rain coats, and hats. "Mushrooms enjoy the rain," said my grandpa. "They will practically come out to throw themselves at our feet in this rain." When it rained at the same time the sun was out, he would call it "mushroom rain." It was a sure sign we'd find lots of mushrooms. We carried big baskets woven out of twigs. Mine was too big for my size. My grandpa carried a stick. First we found wild berries and ate them from the bush as a special meal to "increase our strength." Then we searched for mushrooms. The first mushroom I found looked very beautiful. It had a bright red hat with little white circles and was standing tall and proud, visible from a long distance. I stretched my hand to pick it but my grandfather quickly knocked my hand away, "This is not for us, it's called *muhomor*." I later learned that the common name for this mushroom was fly-agaric, and although this mushroom does not kill people, it has hallucinogenic properties and is used as an aid to travel between the visible and invisible worlds.

My grandfather used his stick to remove the fallen leaves around the trees and to discover small hidden mushrooms we could eat. "The noble mushrooms are hiding," he would say. "You have to use your intuition to find them." He would show me different kinds of mushrooms and tell me their names and uses. This one is good for drying and storing for the winter, this one is delicious pickled, and this one will heal many illnesses.

There is a whole kingdom of mushrooms. Some were used by Gypsies and Russians as food, valued for their high protein content. Some had medicinal use, and some others had psychoactive use. The king of mushrooms is the *Chaga* mushroom, which is very popular in Russia. It is widely used for medicines.

Gypsies collect mushrooms during the late summer and dry them out in the sun on a string where they also absorb the energy of Father Sun. Then it is time to make delicious soup during the winter. Often their very survival depended on how many mushrooms they could gather and dry. You, of course, can purchase fresh or dry mushrooms in a store so there's no excuse not to enjoy them.

Here's a recipe for a wonderful mushroom soup:

Ingredients: One bag of dry mushrooms, one onion, a few potatoes, some carrots, sea salt, pepper, greens (sorrel, parsley) and herbs (dill, sage, dry celery root). Clean and wash the mushrooms (mushrooms are not cleaned and washed before they are dried). Cover them with cold, living water and let them soak for 2-3 hours. Boil the mushrooms in the water used to soak them for 30 minutes. Take the mushrooms out, rinse them with cold, living water, and cut them. Strain the broth. Put the mushrooms back into the broth and add the salt, pepper, and washed, peeled and cut potatoes, carrots, whole onion, and dry celery root. Boil until the potatoes are soft. Discard the onion and celery root. Garnish with chopped fresh greens and herbs.

The mushroom kingdom deserves our respect and admiration. Mushrooms can kill instantly (poisonous) or slowly (candida). Mushrooms can alter the mind instantly (hallucinogenic) or heal slowly (medicinal). The person who knows the secrets of the mushroom kingdom can access parallel worlds, create poison, or cure disease. Anyone who is interested in the kingdom of mushrooms must be very well educated, and it's probably best that you purchase mushrooms only from the most trusted sources. I do not recommend the use of hallucinogenic mushrooms in countries where it's illegal to use them, but if you ever visit a place where they are used in ceremonies, please make sure you are guided by a very experienced and very knowledgeable shaman.

When you start eating living food, drinking living water, and eating nutritious mushrooms that are full of their special sacred energy, you will be naturally "high." You will also be able to have natural visions and intuitive insight during your sleep and in your daydreams as well. You will be plugged into the wisdom of the Kingdom and it will whisper its gentle secrets to you.

Four

RICH IN HEALTH

Good Lessons from Bad Health

Traditionally, Romani people have exceptional health. We say, "A rich man eats well, but God doesn't give him health." This is because rich people tend to eat rich diets and to suffer from that richness.

What does it mean to be healthy? What can we learn when we experience bad health? I'm healthy now, but this wasn't always the case. I've had the good fortune of having bad health at times in my life as well as experiencing vibrant good health. The reason it has been good for me to be sick is that these experiences led me to my life's purpose. I can be trusted to offer solid advice about what it takes to have a healthy and joyful life because I have made that very journey myself.

Years ago I had lost touch with Gypsy ways and had become an unhealthy person. I didn't want to look in the mirror. I would see despair and tears in my eyes. My spine was bent from pain and scoliosis: one shoulder higher, one hip lower. My neck was twisted by muscle spasms. I would habitually stand on one foot because the second one could not bear my weight after an ice skating accident. My face would often be deformed by the pain of severe migraines.

Ten years ago I was in pain most of the time. The pain was so unbearable that on a particularly bad night my husband took me to the emergency room of our local hospital. I remember pleading "Chop my head off!" when I couldn't stand the excruciating pain of this migraine one more second. A doctor with the last name of Paradise—I'm not kidding—gave me a shot that could have put a horse to sleep, yet it wouldn't work for me. I was depressed. I was not healthy, and when I felt the worst, it didn't seem as if life was worth living. On a few occasions I thought seriously about ending my life.

I wasn't always healthy during my childhood either. When I was surrounded by nature at the summer camp for children, I was as strong as the horses I rode bareback. When I was in school in the city, I had chronic sinus infections and my nose would double in size because it was so swollen. It was so bad that I was hospitalized for sinus infections and pain several times. The traditional herbs for healing were not always available, and our diet was poor from lack of nutritious foods in the stores. The doctors decided the only way to cure me was to punch a hole in my sinuses. They tied me to a chair (anesthesia was not used in Russia for such a minor procedure), stuck a long metal needle into one of my nostrils, and pushed. The pain was the worst I have ever felt in my life. I heard a cracking sound and thought that the needle had made a hole in my skull. Blood poured down my chin and flooded my shirt. The procedure didn't work. I kept getting sinus infections. I started getting severe nose bleeds. I was not healthy during winters.

I was also not healthy when I was born. I was worse than not healthy; I was literally dead. My mother told me that the first time she saw me my skin was blue. I didn't breathe and my heart didn't beat. Maybe the doctors saved my life or maybe my mother's prayer saved my life. At different times I've heard she's "hopeless, incurable, no chance, nothing can be done" about some condition or another. I wasn't suffering from anything terminal; I was just always miserable. I was told once that I would spend my life in a wheelchair, and the despair of hearing that almost did the trick of putting me in a wheelchair. During a particularly bad time I swallowed a daily dose of opioids, the most powerful of narcotics. My pill cocktail included sleeping pills and all kinds of prescription and over-the-counter medications. They didn't make me healthy.

I know what it's like to suffer in the body. I had two severe traumatic brain injuries, both of which cracked my skull. There's a beautiful song with the lyric, "There's a crack, a crack in everything. That's how the light gets in." The list of physical complaints I have struggled with include: migraines, neck pain, eye pain, anemia, chronic fatigue, arrhythmia, carpal tunnel syndrome, degenerative disk disease, osteoarthritis, bursitis, tendonitis, astigmatism, poor vision, dry eyes, severe acne, mysterious chronic tooth pain, teeth sensitivity, bleeding gums, nose bleeds, frequent colds and flu, insomnia, indigestion, gastritis, knee pain, sinus infections, and dark moods that would not lift. The doctors trained only in clinical medicine gave me pills and more pills for temporary relief that never addressed the underlying imbalances. What I needed was a cure. I needed strength and health.

I had become acclimated to a more western lifestyle and saw medicine as the only answer. Yet when I was at my physically worst, I cried out in my misery, "I can't live like this. I want to feel like I did as a child in the woods!" When I had suicidal thoughts, I remembered my childhood and what it was like to walk barefoot, to swim in the sea, to eat wild berries, greens, weeds, and flowers. It was when I was living the life of a Gypsy that I was full of robust good health.

How had I lost my health? I had become too rational and had closed the door to the magic of life. I had turned my back on my Romani heritage and left "superstition" behind. I finally understood that, as had been predicted so many times for me, it was my fate to help others heal, but first I had to learn how to heal myself. I had to hit the bottom of the well of deep pain and suffering in order to come home to myself and to the Kingdom. I set out to cure myself of all the diseases and ailments that plagued me. I was determined to eliminate all of them—every single one. I set out on my own journey to find and gather the "cards" of wisdom that I had let scatter in the wind.

Now I stand before the mirror a new person. My posture is straight, my smile is wide, my eyes sparkle. I am almost always—no matter what life throws at me—in a good mood. I very rarely get sick, not even with a cold, not even once a year, or even once in five years. I have no aches or pains. I was able to get my vision back to 20/20. I sleep deeply and wake early and feel completely refreshed and rejuvenated. I have boundless energy. I can hike for five hours nonstop in any weather conditions and at the end of the hike, I still have so much energy that I can jog home.

I recently went to a physician for a checkup and some blood work. The physician studied the results with surprise. "You are the healthiest person I've ever seen! How do you do that?" Well, doctors can provide great benefit when you become injured or have certain illnesses, but many of them don't know what to do in order to help you become deeply healthy. Is the truest health the absence of disease, robust good feeling, or both?

Health is when you wake up with so much energy that you jump out of the bed. Health is when you are so happy that you'd like to hug strangers. Health is experiencing a high level of fitness and mental well-being. I will never again turn my back on the lifestyle of my ancestors. I will always embrace a magical way of living. You have this book in your hands for a reason. Fate has placed you and this information together. So let's explore Romani wisdom and help you achieve true health and real joy.

We say the Roma are rich, not in money but in health. On one of the worst days of my life, my mother came home and said matter-of-factly that she had cancer. I was a teenager and didn't know anything about cancer, but I could see the fear in her eyes and I too became afraid. After her surgery, I was so happy when I was finally allowed to visit her that I bounded into the hospital with a big smile on my face. As I walked from one part of the hospital to another, I noticed that *no one* was smiling. The patients were not smiling, the nurses were not smiling, the doctors were not smiling. The hospital was very quiet, but it wasn't a peaceful sort of quiet. Everyone whispered, and it felt as if the whispering was about secrets and fear and worry and anxiety. When I found my mother, she immediately told me to stop smiling. "Why?" I asked.

"It is not polite. All of these patients are going to die. This is the floor for terminal patients."

If either of us had been in touch with our Gypsy nature at this point, we would have realized that if this was true, it would be even more important for the patients to smile so as to invite the most healing possible into that part of the hospital, or if healing was not possible, to celebrate the bit of life that was left by smiling and enjoying every precious minute.

We can only experience the true joy of life when we accept that we will die. It is this awareness that makes all of life sacred. We must be brave in facing the ways in which our bodies break down and prepare to let the soul go. But I was only a teenager when my mother received the news that she would not live long. I didn't understand anything about death yet. At this point in time, both of us were living an unhealthy life and had lost touch with many of the Gypsy ways.

Even my mother, who was a good healer, had been forced to work so hard and had eaten such bad food for so long that she lacked enthusiasm for life and was clearly heading for death.

I was shocked and terrified that my mother was on the floor with terminal patients. I wanted to talk to my mother's doctor immediately. I ran into the office. The doctor was a kind middle-aged woman. She looked very sad. As soon as I told her my name, the doctor's eyes filled with tears.

At that time in Russia, medical care was free for everyone and doctors were paid less than a janitor in America. Only those who were really passionate about helping patients entered the medical profession. My mother's doctor was a very good doctor; she really cared about my mother and she was worried about me. She felt that there was nothing she could do about the cancer at that point.

My mother decided she only had one chance left. She would use the old Russian Gypsy formula for physical health and pray for the best, and if she had to die, she would die well. She knew she had very little time for anything to work. Her plan consisted of three simple words: hunger, cold, and movement.

The Benefits of Hunger

Since the beginning of time, Gypsies have known that abstaining from food is a powerful cure for illness and disease. Animals and small children will intuitively stop eating as soon as they start feeling sick. Digestion takes a lot of our energy. When we are unwell, all our energy is needed for healing. In many cases, it is unwise to waste our precious energy on digestion.

In this book I use the word *hunger* to mean conscious fasting. Historically, Gypsies may have wanted to use conscious fasting when someone was very sick, but they were forced to fast many times during the year due to lack of food available on the road. Gypsies say, "Romani life is half full, half hungry." As hard as it was for Romanies to go hungry, this contributed to their overall stamina and health.

If you are emotionally and physically healthy, fasting a few times a year will help keep you healthy. Fasting can help you handle stress and will support your body in resisting illnesses.

There are many types of fasting: dry (no water or food), only water, only freshly made juices, fasts that exclude all animal food, fasts that limit the amount of fat you take in, fasts that limit the total number of calories, eating meals made out of one type of fruit, eating only during a certain time of the day, and so on. Most major religions require some type of fasting during special times, and Gypsies too understand that there are both spiritual and physical benefits to going without food or water.

Abstaining from food will cure many minor illnesses and can even cure more serious diseases. The type of fasting will depend on the severity of the disease and how much time the person has "left." And absolutely all fasting is difficult. Not only do you have to deal with physical hunger and all the aches and pains that come with the rapid removal of toxins from your body, but also with the deep emotions that surface each time you try to limit the amount of food you eat. These emotions may include fear, anger, anxiety, doubt, despair, loneliness, and depression. This emotional, psychological, and spiritual part of fasting is usually much more difficult to deal with than the physical aspect of fasting.

The first thing my mother did to face the cancer that had been predicted to be terminal was to go on an eleven day juice fast with the supervision of her doctor. Many good books have been written about the power of fasts. If you plan to do any type of fasting, please read several books and find a health practitioner who has experience supervising fasts before you do anything this aggressive. After the fast, my mother changed her diet completely. She stopped eating foods with no or low energy and we both began eating foods with high energy. They were almost impossible to find, but now it was a matter of life or death that we find them, and so we did.

Don't be afraid of hunger; hunger can be your ally. Letting yourself *feel* hunger is not the same as starving yourself. The longest I ever fasted was an eleven day juice fast as a part of my own deep healing, but now I do frequent short fasts. The first fast I did was extremely difficult; then it got easier and easier. You'll know you have exceptional health when fasting is no longer a big deal to you.

Healing With Cold

"Scared of hunger and cold, don't be born a Gypsy." My mother started every day of her healing regimen by filling a big bucket with ice-cold water and pouring it on herself standing in the bathtub. There's a verb in the Russian language that I can't translate properly into English. The approximate translation has the meaning "to increase the body's resistance to disease by exposing the body to cold temperatures." The closest translation to this idea in English is "to temper the body with cold."

During their travels for almost two thousand years, Gypsies became accustomed to spending a lot of time outside during any weather. Gypsies would walk barefoot even during the winter. Now, when I walk barefoot in the snow, people look at me as if I have lost my mind. And I'm always smiling when I do it, which probably makes them even more suspicious. If only they knew that this is the best method to build resistance to colds, they would take off their shoes and socks and would walk along with me.

Roma say, "Let an old man buy fur coat and felt boots; I'll do very well without them." Which means he won't live long anyway, but I will if I expose myself to the cold.

Many Russians know of the famous Russian healer Porfiry Ivanov. Porfiry was born in 1898 in a small village. He wasn't any different from his neighbors. At the age of thirty-five, he found out that he had the last stage of cancer. Nothing could be done. Porfiry was in a lot of pain that couldn't be helped with any medication. In an act of desperation, he decided to kill himself. During a bitter cold winter, he undressed and jumped into a river that was mostly covered with ice. He didn't drown, so he came out of the river and decided to stand outside, wet, with no clothes, so that he could catch pneumonia and die from that. He stood there, freezing, for several hours, and then he went home. In the morning, he woke up feeling just fine, so he repeated the same "procedure" and jumped in the water and stood in the cold. After a month of this treatment, he had cured himself. In a while, he began teaching others to use cold for healing and became known in Russia and Ukraine simply as Teacher. If you ever see pictures of Porfiry, you will notice that in every single photograph he wears nothing but shorts. For the next fifty years he would walk only in shorts, barefoot, during any season and any weather.

If you would like to use the healing power of cold, start slowly. In the morning, wash your face with cold water, and in the evening, stand in a shallow bathtub of very cold water for several seconds. Get in the habit of finishing a hot shower with several seconds of cold water. Gradually and very slowly increase the time you expose yourself to cold water. Then pour a bucket of ice cold water on yourself, outside if you have a back-yard. During the summer, start walking outside barefoot for several minutes. As the fall takes over the summer, keep walking barefoot. During the winter, run at least several leaps in the snow barefoot. If you are doing it right, you will feel incredible internal heat and full of energy.

Once there lived a wicked old woman who had her own daughter, Marfusha, and a step-daughter, Nastenka. Marfusha did nothing around the house; Nastenka did all the work. Still, the stepmother found fault in everything she did. When Nastenka was bringing buckets of water to the house, young men would stop to admire her. No one noticed Marfusha. So, one winter day, the stepmother decided to get rid of Nastenka. She ordered her husband, "Take this nasty girl deep into the forest, so that my eyes no longer have to see her, so that my ears no longer have to hear her. Leave her there, to die in the bitter cold."

"Have you lost your mind?" yelled the old man.

"Take her to the woods. If you don't follow my order, I will throw you both out!" Even a hurricane will calm down, but a wicked woman will not. The old man could do nothing else. He grieved and wept but put his daughter into the sled, took her deep into the forest, and left her there.

Nastenka sat down right on the snow, her body shivering and her teeth chattering. All of a sudden, Grandpa

Frost came in his sled pulled by three beautiful white horses. He saw Nastenka, and how pale she was. She had a thin coat, light boots, and no mittens. "Are you warm, young lady?" he asked. "Yes, Grandpa," she replied, "I am warm." Hearing these words, Grandpa Frost ran around Nastenka, making it even colder. "Are you warm now?" he asked. "Yes, Grandpa, thank you, I am warm," said Nastenka, although her lips were blue and barely moved from bitter cold. Grandpa Frost smiled, "I see you are not afraid of me. That deserves a reward!" He took his fur coat off and wrapped it around Nastenka's shoulders; she instantly felt warm. "Take my sled with my horses and here," he clapped his hands and a big chest appeared in the sled, "are some gifts for your family." Nastenka sat on the sled and the horses danced, their bells making a joyful sound as they approached the village.

Men, women, and children ran after the sled, following it to Nastenka's house. The stepmother, Marfusha, and the old man came out to see what was going on. Nastenka stepped down from the sled, "Please don't be angry, Mother, I brought you some gifts from Grandpa Frost." She opened the chest and everyone gasped: it was filled with sparkling jewelry and gold.

The stepmother couldn't hide her jealousy. "Take Marfusha to the same spot," she ordered her husband. The old man took Marfusha deep into the forest and left her with a basket full of food. Marfusha had a thick blanket to sit on, a fur coat, warm boots, and wool mittens. She was eating pastry after pastry when Grandpa Frost appeared. "Are you warm, young lady?" he asked. "Are you blind, disgusting old man?" she yelled, "Can't you see that I am cold, very cold?" Hearing these words, Grandpa Frost ran around Marfusha, making it even colder. "Are you warm now?" he asked. "Hey, old man," said Marfusha, "give me your sled, your horses, and a big chest full of jewelry and gold. And hurry. I don't want to freeze here!"

The stepmother was waiting in the porch when the sled with Marfusha appeared. Men, women, and children were running after the sled, laughing. You see, it wasn't pulled by three beautiful horses; it was pulled by three pigs. When the sled stopped at the house, the stepmother ran to open the big chest and then hastened out of the way. A dozen crows flew out of it. The stepmother and Marfusha ran inside the house, ashamed.

Soon, Nastenka married a handsome and kind young man. I was invited to their wedding. The tables were heavy with delicious food but I didn't eat much; I was busy staring at the happy couple.

Move and Live

To try to save herself from cancer, my mother would go outside every single day, even if it was windy, raining, or snowing. She was very weak at first, so she could not walk very far. But every day she would add a few more minutes until she could walk for hours.

What happened to my mother? In time she felt so good that if the cancer had not been cured and she would have died, she at least would have died happy. But what happened instead was that her doctors were amazed to discover that the cancer they thought would kill her was gone. My mother had healed herself with hunger, cold, and movement. She had healed herself with good food and joy and an appreciation for her life. It took coming to the brink of death for my mother to change her life, but she did it.

Not only was she able to cure herself from cancer, but her severe allergies and phobia of closed spaces were gone too. My mother had been allergic to just about everything that grew: raw vegetables, flowers, trees, and grasses. When I was a child, she would peel some carrots and potatoes for the soup and sneeze non-stop. Tears would keep rolling down her cheeks. The same would happen if she went outside during the spring. As a side benefit to the work she did to cure her cancer, her allergies were gone. My mother also used to experience panic any time she was in a closed space, such as an elevator or a bus. Her doctor had prescribed medication to calm her down that was highly addictive and made her feel unwell. With her new robust physical health, her mind and spirit were also healthy and this phobia was now also gone.

I've shared the story of my mother's healing to show you that big, miraculous things are possible. I received a call recently from a client sharing a story that will help you see that the practical application of these principles in everyday life also works brilliantly in circumstances that are less dire. My client was a relatively healthy woman who was accustomed to having a medicine cabinet full of remedies for what she thought of as small things. Like many people, she used a combination of prescribed medicines, over-the-counter medications, herbal and other remedies. She suffered occasional migraines and allergies during "allergy season", and she regularly put up with menstrual cramps, motion sickness, and insomnia. She also thought it was normal to have a couple of colds every year and the flu every couple of years.

A few years ago when she was going through a divorce and was depressed and feeling tired and unhealthy, she consulted with me about cleaning up all aspects of her life. She trusted the advice I gave her about Gypsy wisdom and adopted all of the practices that I am now sharing with you. Without trying, she lost weight. She gained tremendous energy and enthusiasm for life. She feels creative and empowered, and her overall health has improved so that the small illnesses and health problems she was working around have completely been resolved. Her relationships are better. Her life force is strong. She is so comfortable living a healthy life that she has even forgotten what it was like to have any sort of health problem. She remembered recently when she was dusting off the medicine box in the back of a bathroom shelf and discovered all sorts of pills with past expiration dates. Pills and remedies she hasn't needed or used in years. When she filled out a medical form recently, she answered the question *What medications do you take regularly?* with this answer: None. Not even one!

Stop eating even when you know you could eat more but are aware that you are fully nourished. Walk outside every day and look for opportunities to sit in the sun for a moment. Splash some cold water on yourself whenever you can. The writer D. H. Lawrence wrote, "When we get out of the glass bottle of our ego, and when we escape like the squirrels in the cages of our personality and get into the forest again, we shall shiver with cold and fright but things will happen to us so that we don't know ourselves. Cool, unlying life will rush in." Let life in! Make yourself uncomfortable to find a deeper experience of the world and your place in it.

Make sure you add more extremes to your rituals of how you take care of yourself. There should be balance between being hungry and too full, moving until exhaustion and not moving at all, being cold and spending all your time in heated rooms. When you find this balance—not in the soft middle but more on the edges of your physical experience—you'll experience robust health.

Challenge yourself to get healthy and stay healthy now, rather than facing a serious disease later. A strong foundation of health will give you a longer and stronger life. If you wait until you've abused your body and have an illness or disease, you'll have to change your life by almost being frightened to death. I'd rather have you singing and dancing in good health through every age of your life than having to get sick to be sober about how important it is to take care of yourself properly. Gypsy wisdom is very simple, and once you grasp it and live it you won't revert back to your bad old ways because you'll be too joyful in your new life to move backward. If you slip a little bit, you'll feel the difference and will return to a whole and healthy life.

Problem: Having no energy, feeling tired most of the time.
Solution: Wash your face and hands with very cold water (as cold as it gets from your faucet). Pour some very cold water in a bucket and stand in it for thirty seconds. End each hot shower with several seconds of a very cold shower. Get as much fresh air and sunshine as you can. Stop eating and drinking several hours before going to bed: you will wake up with much more energy.

Problem: Insomnia.
Solution: Start walking outside as much as you can. Start with ten minute walks several times a day. Increase to thirty minute walks. Roma say, "If all you do all day is walk, you'll sleep like a log."

Problem: "Restless leg syndrome"
Solution: Educate yourself on the benefits of Magnesium supplement and Marjoram essential oil. And then listen to your legs! They are restless for a reason. If you drive to work, sit all day, and watch television all night, your legs will scream at you, "Please do something! Take a walk. Dance, for heaven's sake!" At the very least when you are in bed trying to sleep and can't because your legs are "restless", plant your heels, raise your toes, and vigorously move your feet from side to side for five or ten minutes. This will release the pent up energy of your legs. But to make them really happy, they need to move and dance, and so do you.

Gypsies dance at any opportunity we get. If you look on the internet for Gypsies dancing you'll find some wonderful examples. We just jump in at any age and with any excuse to dance. It's Wednesday? What a perfect time to dance. Just lost your job? Better round up some friends, have a party, and dance!

Find a type of movement that gives you joy, and then your passion for it will become a part of your life. Jumping on a trampoline, taking dance lessons, playing a sport, riding a bike, something you find freeing and fulfilling. Move like a child: be silly, roll down a grassy hill (when was the last time you rolled down a hill covered with green, soft grass?), jump up and down, jog and make funny faces at the same time. I just saw a grandmother running barefoot in the stream in a city park. I couldn't tell who was having more fun: the grandmother or the granddaughter!

A quarter of the American population doesn't exercise at all (meaning not even walking or gardening). To really live, you have to move your body every single day.

There lived a vicious duke near where I was traveling. More than anything he hated Gypsies. He would not leave them alone. Gypsies made a camp in his forest and he demanded gold coins in return. Where would Roma find even a silver coin, let alone a gold coin? So the duke demanded they give him their horses. How will Rom live without a horse? "And if you don't give me your horses today, I will take them by force myself tomorrow," said the duke. Then Shuvihano went deep into the forest and appealed to Veshitko Dad for help. "The duke is rolling in money but will not rest until there are no horses left in our taboro. Help us, Veshitko Dad, advise us what to do." Replies Veshitko Dad, "You see a branch on the ground? It is not a simple branch, it is magical. Make a pipe out of it. Next time the duke appears in your camp, start playing the pipe. The duke will start dancing and will keep dancing until you stop playing the pipe." With that said, Veshitko Dad vanished into thin air.

Shuvihano picked up the branch, made a pipe. and went back to the camp. Soon the duke galloped into camp along with his armed servants. He jumped off his horse and was very pleased with himself, "Your horses are my horses now!" At this very moment, Shuvihano began playing the pipe. The duke awkwardly moved his shoulders up and down, twisted his body left and right, and began dancing. The whole taboro gathered to see what was going on. Look at him squatting and jumping, turning and bending, slapping his sides, not being able to stop. Shuvihano is playing the pipe; the duke is dancing. Finally the duke begged, "Rom, stop playing the pipe, I can no longer dance!" But Shuvihano didn't turn a hair. He played the pipe, amusing everyone in the taboro, for their joy, for the duke's grief. "Rom, Rom, ask for anything you wish, I will fulfill it, only stop playing the pipe!"

"All right, I will stop. But give me your word that you will not plot against us and will leave us alone."

The duke gave him his word. Shuvihano stopped playing the pipe and the duke collapsed in a heap on the ground. People say that from that time the duke became kind and sweet-tempered. He wouldn't hurt a soul and helped anyone in need. Last I heard he left his castle and joined the Gypsies.

Healing in The Trees

One of my favorite things to do is read medical studies. Perhaps I do it so you don't have to. I often smile happily to myself as I learn that researchers at respected institutions in laboratories wearing white coats, gathering data, and engaging in experiments "discover" miraculous "new" findings like this.

Researchers in Japan are studying the positive benefits of spending time in the woods and have found that it lowers the levels of cortisol, the hormone that rises when we're under stress and is the root of many serious illnesses. Spending time with trees also lowers blood pressure and pulse rate and triggers a dramatic increase in the activity of NK, or "natural killer" cells, which are produced by the immune system to ward off infection and fight cancer.

A large-scale study at the University of Michigan created a research partnership with three respected universities in the U.K. and worked together to evaluate 1,991 individuals who walked with a group in nature at least once a week. Will their findings surprise you at this point, or will you join me in smiling with delight? They found...wait for it...that connecting with nature provides a measurable psychological lift, significantly lowers the risk for depression, lessens stress, and enhances one's sense of well-being. But wait, there's more. Walkers in rural areas reported less stress, less negativity, and greater well-being than those who walked on city streets. And people who had recently experienced stressful life events such as a serious illness, divorce, unemployment, or death of a loved one especially benefited from the outdoor group walks. Not on a treadmill, pounding away in a gym with bad news blaring on large televisions hanging everywhere. Not alone. In nature. In a group. Sounds like my taboro. I wish they had called it the Gypsy Study.

Five

GATHER AROUND THE FIRE

Burning Brightly

It is said that Gypsies always get along with fire and that Romanies know spells to protect from fire—meaning that Gypsies never cause a forest or house fire. We love fire and know that a prayer delivered next to a fire will rise with the smoke and that messages from God can also be received when the hands are stretched out to the cracking warmth of a fire.

Fire is healing and cleansing; it provides inspiration, burns problems away, and creates unity between people when they gather. Do you have some fire in your life? Can you gather around a fire pit in the backyard, a campfire, or around a fireplace with people you love very soon? Singing songs and dancing near a fire, and making food on a fire are very spiritual experiences.

To prepare a simple dish of "Potatoes Out Of A Fire," burn a fire down until there are just hot coals at a time when you are hungry and will appreciate the food more. Bury the potatoes with the skins on (but no tin foil) under the hot coals and ash and leave them there for 45 minutes while you tell stories, sing, and enjoy the company of family and friends. Use a stick to lift the potatoes out and cool them by quickly, throwing them from hand to hand. You won't get burned if you do it quickly. Dust off the ashes and eat your potato with a little sea salt or salt from high in the mountains. A simple potato cooked this way can taste like the food of the Gods. It will remind you of the simple bounty of the Earth.

Try this. Walk away from a fire during the winter, let yourself feel the cold, and then warm up by the fire again. Put your hands into the snow and keep them there until you feel the burning sensation from the cold. Shake off the snow and place your hands next to the fire. You will feel very strong heat coming from inside of you, and yet you will not feel hot. The coldness of the snow will feel hotter than the heat from the fire, and you will see steam rising from your palms and fingers. It's quite a sight! Your hands are almost on fire but you feel pleasant. No words can describe it, you just have to try it. The stars will smile at you and all of your senses will be heightened. Your intuition will be heightened too.

Fire is the source of great energy, strength, and stamina. It will give you wonderful dreams, create deep friendships, support your family and friends, and open your heart. A fire teaches hospitality and kindness. It is said to attract the little people and spirits of the forest. The shadows the fire casts can become the theatre of the imagination. We say, "Gypsies learn their destiny from the fire." Perhaps you'll find your destiny looking quietly at a fire and asking for the answers you seek.

The New Campfire

We spend more and more time in the artificial world made of houses, offices, stores, and cars. We spend more and more time *inside* and unconnected to the life force of the Universe. We think we don't have time to walk outside, or enjoy the good health of our bodies, or attend to our spirits, and yet we seem to have plenty of time to watch TV! The average American home has more televisions than people. The average American watches over 4 hours and 35 minutes of television *every day*. I'll save you the math—that's 32 hours per week, 140 hours a month, which is a shocking nearly six complete days in front of the television every month, and almost 72 days in just one year. I absolutely refuse to calculate the time spent watching television over the average lifespan because that number would break my heart. What on Earth are we doing?

Entertainment and information are important parts of life, and we get a great deal that is positive from television and the internet, but let me tell you as a Gypsy, you had better watch only what you feel *passionate* about and not waste time on anything else. Television and the internet are not a substitute for relationships with your family and friends or a connection to nature or a replacement for romance. Time spent passively taking in too much harmful information, playing virtual games, or exposing yourself to sloppy entertainment that doesn't really excite you will drain your energy and harm your overall health.

Imagine the television and the internet as the modern equivalent of ancient fires. These are places we can very intentionally gather around to hear stories and connect with others, but don't make them a substitute for a real fire and real relationships. Connect with people who are close to you to share information and stories, attend movies, watch television together, and enjoy social networking websites. But make certain that the time you spend in this way is chosen consciously and is *adding* something to your life. Feed your soul and your connection to others and nature as your first priority.

If television and the internet are not carefully controlled, you can waste your life force and distract yourself from what matters most for literally weeks, months, and years at a time. Turn on something when you absolutely love it and feel great enthusiasm for it, and when you don't, please turn it off!

Six

Lucky In Love

New Love the Old Way

The Gypsy wisdom I'm going to share with you about relationships may seem very old fashioned, but I invite you to begin exploring these ideas with an open mind and set aside what you know about how things commonly work in our modern world. For just a few minutes, take on a new way to experience ideas about marriage and family—just for the time you read this--and see how it feels to you. Rather than being "out of date", you may find that these ideas about love seem progressive, modern, even revolutionary.

Gypsy people who love their culture don't shift with the changing winds, they hold fast to things that provide the greatest benefit for the most people over the longest period of time. For this reason, very little has changed in the way relationships between men and women work in the Romani way. There is no casual dating. There is no trying people on and having sex with them and dropping them after using them for a short time. No casual sex for the "fun" of it. No light talk amongst women and men that they can be collected as playthings. No glorifying the man who is the "player." We understand that marriage and the decision to have children will have long-lasting consequences on our own health and well-being, the level of our lasting happiness, what our family is able to focus on, and the general well-being of our community.

A good match that is solid over time and is happy overall contributes to the stability and peace of the extended family and the entire taboro. A child conceived by a couple who have committed to be together and whose families are backing them up in that commitment will be a child who is wanted and surrounded with support even before birth.

A tempestuous and broken relationship causes great pain, not just to the couple who suffers the drama, but to everyone around them. For this reason it is thought that people should have help choosing each other and that the parents and the larger community should have a say in this magical process.

It may seem like true freedom to make all of your choices and be with whomever you want whenever you want, but that so-called freedom can really be self indulgent or reckless. Here's something Gypsies understand well. Sexual connection creates bonds between people at an energetic level and this linking of people needs to be done very carefully. Once the chemical bonding of lovers takes hold, they both don't think clearly anymore and can make mistakes about who to be with long-term. As a result, we Romani keep men and women separated in many situations and go about creating connections between them slowly and carefully. Love, commitment, and lasting relationships are very important--too important to take lightly. We don't want to be sloppy or make a mess out of the potential for marriage. Too much is at stake.

Traditionally, parents carefully discuss, plan, and at some level arrange the marriages, or the meetings between people who are seen as having good marriage potential for each other, to help nature along in a certain healthy direction. It is not allowed that couples have sex before they are married. Now things have softened a bit, but young people are still more inclined to follow the advice of their parents in Romani society than in the rest of society. The wisdom of parents and grandparents is seen as very valuable, and young people listen respectfully to the wisdom of older generations.

Families considering becoming linked by marriage size each other up carefully. Do we want to spend the rest of our lives eating meals with these people? If this couple marries, what will sharing grandchildren be like? Who are these people at their core and can we embrace them? What about this particular man and woman would make a good marriage? Where would it be challenging, perhaps too challenging, to be a good match? Do they have the right things in common? Is there a spark between them? What would the personality of the marriage be with these two coming together? Divinations are also used to help the process along.

You see the parents of the groom watching a prospective bride with great care. How does this young women interact with others, what actions and words reveal her true character? Is she good natured, is she kind, hard-working, patient, fun? Would she be a loving and affectionate wife to our son and a good mother to their children? Families look for signs that she's naturally happy. Does she sing and dance? Is there a spring in her step and a glimmer in her eye? They want their son to have good company on the journey of life.

You see the parents of a girl who is ready to be a bride watching a prospective groom and sizing him up over time. Who are his friends? Is he quick to anger? What choices does he make on a daily basis? Is he hard-working without complaint? Is he protective? Does he put others first? Will he be there for her and for their children? Can he handle life with courage? Will he enjoy being a strong husband and father?

If you'd like, you can take a look back at your own romantic history. Did your friends warn you that they didn't think you had chosen wisely but you went forward anyway with a negative result? Assuming that your parents and grandparents and your aunts and uncles know you well and adore you—would they have picked the partner you chose or would they have directed you in another way?

We've all experienced the pain of a wedding that's an ill-fated match from the beginning where everyone just knows there isn't a chance the marriage will be happy and last, and yet no one says anything early on or asks to be consulted. The guests are speculating on how long it will take for the relationship to blow apart but outwardly are forcing smiles and sharing best wishes as they hand over the gift of a casserole dish that very may well be thrown across the room by the bride or groom on some dark and stormy night.

Now contrast that with this experience. Have you ever been to a wedding that's a blessed match and everyone knows it? This is a real marriage and a cause for real celebration. There's magic in the air. If little things go wrong on the big day, no one minds because what matters is the joining of lives and families with true joy. It's fun. The dancing is real. The food tastes better. The laughter is genuine. The stories flow. The music feels just right. This is a wedding a community of friends and family can get behind. This is a match where the couple will continue to seek support and advice from elders to keep their union strong. It's not just an expensive party with cake, it's a real marriage, and that's a cause for celebration!

Men Are Men, Women Are Women

In a Gypsy family, the women genuinely respect and honor the men. And the men must treat the women in a cherishing and loving way that recognizes their importance. Does the difference between men and women matter? In our world today, there are fewer distinctions between men and women and their roles and responsibilities, but in Romani life the differences are cultivated so that masculinity is prized and a woman who is poised and feminine gives those gifts to her family and the taboro. Who they are together as a couple must make a valuable contribution, and the differences between them are what creates the spark in their union.

Women and men are separate much of the time. Women spend time with women, talking and supporting each other and working things out together. Women process their emotions and tell their stories to each other and get the support they need rather than talking their men to death.

And men spend time with men addressing their concerns, using their friendships and family relationships to hold each other accountable and build the community. Men make each other behave and keep each other accountable, and this frees women to relax and enjoy their men.

Do you see the value in this? When the genders first spend time in their own groups and then come together to spend time as a couple, they are refreshed, supported, and prepared to be together. They don't wear each other out with the things that are believed to be best handled in other ways. They can be the best they can to each other. The romance and passion are alive.

When I see a husband dutifully carrying his wife's purse as he follows along as she shops, I'm tempted to pull her aside and whisper: *A man who is a lap dog is not a happy man and a woman with a lapdog would really rather have a real man. Wouldn't you rather your husband be with men right now doing "manly things" so that when you come home and show him the lovely thing you just bought he can see you in a delicious new way and fall in love with you again?*

When I see a woman who clearly isn't at all interested in the sporting event she is gritting her teeth through beside her husband,

I feel like whispering in his ear: *What if you enjoyed this game with your buddies, amped up your testosterone, and returned to your wife who had spent a relaxed afternoon with her sisters and girlfriends, getting a massage and being in nature? The sparks would fly all night!*

Sometimes the "together" time a couple spends doesn't create more intimacy, but less. Think about the way you spend time with your partner. Are there ways to give yourself a bit more breathing room to be a man and a woman that would enhance your relationship? The differences between us are to be prized and loved. The elders in my taboro taught me this.

What the Old Ones Know

The most status in a Romani family belongs to the oldest woman of the family. The word of the oldest woman is law. It is recognized that she will be the wisest person in the whole community. She is respected and admired.

Traditionally, the women of the family hold it together, get up early, use gifts they may have for fortune-telling, go to the market, buy food, and then prepare the food and serve it to the family. Women in a traditional Gypsy family have the status of provider and nurturer. Because of the historical discrimination against Gypsies for so many generations, it may have been more difficult for men to make money. It still may be harder for them to be hired for work. It's interesting to me that men traditionally don't do fortune-telling (I've seen exceptions in modern life). But it is men who hold the larger community together, and they are the ones who dictate the laws. They are in charge of the community and keeping the Gypsy culture alive. Young men are mentored by old men. They learn how to be good men by spending time with the natural leaders of the taboro. There are many rules in the Gypsy culture that have to be followed, and holding everyone to this standard is the work of the men. Men make sure everyone knows the rules. They have their own court to solve problems within the group. A Gypsy community is bound together very tightly.

Traditionally, men cared for animals and traded horses, and today they often find work selling cars or working on them, but usually it is the women who take care of the family and the men who link the family to the community. Women have power, but they don't brag about it or hold it over the heads of men. From what outsiders see, they might think that men have all power and respect in the family, but really it is the women who hold it all together and the men who protect it and expand it into the larger community. This is the wisdom that has been handed down to us by our elders.

We Are Everything to Each Other

The passionate connection between a man and wife is very private in Gypsy culture, but it is also seen as the most important thing. The ideal is that a husband thinks of his wife as a prize he treasures, and that she thinks of him as the best of everything.

The Romani people also value the bond with their children as much as their marriage. Any separation between a couple and their children just doesn't make sense. You hand your children over to someone else to raise? You spend time in separate rooms at night, all watching different entertainment on different screens? You barely speak to each other, or you speak harshly to each other? You come home late because you care more about being at the office earning money than being with your *family*? These ways of being seem absolutely crazy to a Gypsy.

The love and connection of a family and the love between a husband and wife that spills over to their children is the most important thing in the world. Protecting the family and making sure that the family is happy and that everyone has their basic physical needs met and all of their emotional needs met are the top priorities. Love is absolutely at the center of life. The Romani love their children with devotion, and this is a source of status in the culture. Families that don't get along don't have the same status as families that get along well. Marriages that are strong and where there is no cheating or even looking at anyone else are marriages that are deeply respected and convey high status in Gypsy culture.

Couples look after themselves and their children, then the extended family and the community. Everything else in life is far below those essential priorities. Women make sure that their families are strong and happy. If there is vibrancy and passion in relationships, then all is right with the world. Emotions are expressed with the men being bold and laughing loudly and women letting their emotions fly around the room, out the window, and up into the branches of a tree. Gypsies don't hold back.

Now how does all or any of this apply to you? That's up to you to consider, but here's something you can do if you choose. Take a moment with a piece of paper and a nice pen and something delicious to drink, and I hope by now you know I'm going to suggest you be outside under a big tree or near water. Now that you've established some peace and quiet, think of the ways your family may not be getting the best of you and what you could do to change that. How can you be more passionate in your marriage? If you aren't married but want to be, how can you create a connection that is full of passion and vibrancy and that is at the center of your world? Who loves you the most that you can ask for help finding your right partner? If you have children, how can you make them your absolute top priority? How can things shift in your life to put spending joyful time with your children as the most important thing on your to-do list? How are you connecting to your chosen community? Do you spend enough time with people of your own gender so that you are fed by that energy and can bring your best to your partner? What priority is given to the couples and children in your extended family? Do they receive material things or precious time from you? Are you making memories by engaging in meaningful activities together? Do you create experiences that are memorable and build your joy and connection as a family, or are you wasting precious hours with passive viewing of entertainment that adds up to nothing being done, created, or built? We are most alive in our families and communities. How can you shine more light and more love on the people around you? What can you do to actively bring greater love into your life?

Private Romance—We Don't Say Sex

Romani are private people and our rules about the body and sex are things that are shared quietly, respectfully, and not discussed openly. I've wondered if I should even write about this, and in the end I decided to share some things which you may find useful. After all, every single one of my clients comes to me first to get help in relationships and only then in health. At the heart of our laws about dress, taking care of the body, and our rules about "private romance" is the underlying reverence we feel for our bodies. It's not prudishness by any stretch of the imagination. In fact, I think our ways help preserve the special sexual energy between people.

Women use one towel for their lower body and feet and another for the upper body. Our strict rules about cleanliness have been with us for thousands of years—long before the link between germs and illness was commonly understood. Following these strict rules has contributed to our robust good health through many generations.

We love our bodies and care for them with reverence so that we can bring our best to each other.

How you move and how you care for yourself every day is very important. How you dress and take care of the smallest details of your nails and hair shows that you care about yourself and your partner. Your home must be absolutely clean and orderly and smell great and look delightful to the eye. You must care for your body in ways that stimulate your senses and celebrate the joy of living inside your own skin.

Sing to music in the car. Create your work space so that it is exciting. While you are engaged in what you love, your soul must be fed. Wear clothes that make you feel incredibly attractive. Love the people with whom you work and be open with your friends and family so that they know your true heart. When your entire life is based on love and enthusiasm, you will notice the sun going down with delight. It's time! You will make love as a fulfilled and happy person who is literally full of life and the beautiful feelings within you.

Your evening meal can be a love potion. Experiment with the magical power of nature around you and in you, and mix your experiences and your unique imagination to create an elixir for living and loving in all of your actions.

Traditional Gypsy women do not wear skirts shorter than knee-length, and there is a very good reason for this. How we are in private is different than how we are in public. We save our most sexual side for the man in our life and don't put our sexuality on cheap display. This isn't to say that we aren't sexy in the way we dress. Romani women love to show the shape of their bodies in their clothes and to dress in flowing fabrics of beautiful colors. There is just a fine line between feminine seduction that leaves some things to the imagination and something that feels tasteless.

Gypsy women don't want to dress in a masculine way and imitate men. We want to celebrate our femininity and have them show us their masculinity. We want a man to open the top buttons of his shirt to show a chest that is muscled. We want men to embrace their strength and power, to stand tall and proud.

The art of seduction is a true dance between the sun and the moon, the masculine and the feminine. It's the polarity that is juicy and exciting. Flamenco comes from Gypsy culture. In this dance, the man is straightforward; he shows what he is made of, his manliness, determination, strength, his presence, all on proud display. The woman shows the lines of her body, throws her head back, and is dressed beautifully. Her femininity, her power, and her sexuality are clear, and with the clapping of her hands and the stamping of her feet, you can see that she demands a good man in order to open herself up. A woman like that won't take just anyone.

This dance is an eloquent conversation without words about who you are and who I am. As we dance, we show each other who we are and we flirt and seduce at a level that has great magnetism.

The dance of the woman twirling her skirt suggests: *Come closer, and then I may choose to come closer to you, or perhaps I'll move away from you. You can only have me if you are worthy of me. See if you think you are worthy of me.*

And the dance of the man communicates: *I may want you right here and right now and I need you, or maybe I don't need you, and I'm fine by myself—but oh, you are so beautiful I probably won't be able to resist you.*

This is the intricate dance of attraction and connection. It can be playful. It can be intense. It can feel dangerous. It can feel safe. This level of erotic engagement is not just for courtship and mating--it is for a lifetime if a couple wants their relationship to remain strong.

As soon as this beautiful dance between them stops, the relationship dies. And so Gypsies dance until the end of life, and you can use your imagination to understand what that means.

In Nature as God and Goddess

A key element to a successful union is not just having sex, but making love in a way that moves beyond the physical into the spiritual and magical realms where time stops. When a man and woman love and trust each other, they are free to be wildly passionate and explore whatever they want to explore together and to be fully there for each other.

What could possibly be more important than a mystical union and the art of lovemaking so that the two truly become ONE? This desire goes beyond merely physical desire to the desire to connect through one's mate with the entire world and the Universe. When this level of connection is present there is no desire to seek someone else because the union fills a couple up to the brim. People seek others in affairs when their emotional, mental, physical, and spiritual needs aren't met in the way they take care of themselves as individuals and how they take care of themselves as a couple. To have a powerful spark with someone else you must first have it within yourself. To have it within your connection to the special one in your bed you must not share that magical energy beyond that sacred bed.

You cannot be so tired and crushed by the routine of your life that you come home from work that you hate, eat bad food, and take your partner for granted. Deep loving is about meeting each other as a God and Goddess. Preparing for each other in ways that make time together special is an art and science. Understanding what is required of you to be a great partner is the first thing to master.

Open your eyes and smile at your beloved because you are welcoming the vitality of the day into the magic of the night. Make love with inspiration. Live in the body and spirit from morning to night in order to make love in a way that is worthy of you and your partner. You will know you have made magical love when you fall into shared dreams throughout the night together. When your bodies stay entwined after you make love and your sleep is so deep that you are as rested as if you've had a vacation. That's when you'll know you're bringing your best to each other.

The magic of sex is not to be found in grabbing at each other in the dark to seek quick release. It is being fully present to your own life and being grateful that you have someone wonderful to share your body and life with so that you want to dive into them with great passion and desire and love.

Great love is about appreciating the beauty and handsomeness in each other. Seeing the soul of the other. Expressing fully and with joy. You can't "make love" if you are unloving and unhappy. You can't be unsatisfied and unfulfilled in your life and have great sex. To be a wonderful lover you must first be a wonderful lover to yourself.

Playfulness and freedom comes when we are feeling great and when we cultivate our passion and share it freely with our partner. Sex is not a sleeping pill. Flat energy in bed is not what we were made to experience. What celebrates the body celebrates the senses of taste, smell, sight, touch, and the depths of the unseen world of intuition. Making love is a magical art. How do you use your senses when you make love? What do you do to thoughtfully set the stage for your lovemaking in your bedroom, or in the woods? Before you can really deeply fall in love with a person, you must fall in love with life and nature, because there is nothing that will bring more of nature to you than being sexual with the one you love in a way that is earthy and rich and grounded in what it means to be alive.

Real Love Is Real

I've had clients who were single and stuck in fantasies about the perfect person they imagined would love them. They dated and had a few months of passion out of the magic of being in love and then ended it and moved on quickly when the "magic" seemed to fade. I've worked with these clients to help them become less brittle and judgmental and to be more fluid and earthy in their approach to love.

Real relationships are imperfect because we are all imperfect. To go deep we must be courageous about what we will find at the bottom of the lake when we go into deeper things. Hurt will be stirred up in the mud on the bottom of the lake. Difficulties will come, and to sustain a lasting love you must sustain the qualities of love in general in every aspect of your life and the way you love each other.

I'm not going to teach you Gypsy love charms and potions directed at a specific person to fall in love with you because you don't want anyone to be coerced to love you, and you don't want love to come to you in that way either. How would you feel if you were manipulated into caring for someone, but the charm's power dissipated and then there wasn't any substance underneath it? Don't force someone and in return you won't be forced. Choose freely and with open eyes. And when you know you have someone you can deeply love, create your own rituals to strengthen the magic between you so that it lasts and lasts. You can even use the very special essential oils mentioned at the end of the book to create these rituals.

This is much more than playing "our song"; it is the rich language, symbols, and rituals that a thoughtful man and woman shape together over time. The language only you two understand.

Love Rituals

I enjoy teaching my clients things like an old Gypsy charm of tying a knot in each others' hair to bind love together. And one of my favorite things to have couples do is to create a special box to keep their love safe. Seal your emotional connection and make the bond between you stronger by creating a safe and beautiful place to hold your love.

When you enjoy a place and time together, pick up a pebble or an acorn and give it to your beloved as a gift to signify where you were and what you found beautiful in that moment. Place a shell from the beach that beautiful afternoon you spent in deep conversation in your special box. Give each other jewelry—it doesn't have to be expensive—but it does need to have symbolic importance and matter to you. Save the ticket stubs from special events together. Create a treasure trove of memories.

You are creating a physical manifestation of your love. Outgrow your box over the years as you fill it with letters, cards, objects, symbols, anything that has meaning and is an expression of your love for each other. Keep your box in a special place in your bedroom. When you have difficulties--and you will--each of you can go to the box to remember where you have been and what you have created together. Reconnect with who you are and who they are and help yourself fall in love with them over and over again.

I hope you outgrow your box on a regular basis and that at the end of your life it will be a huge trunkful of memories and connections. These will be private things, passionate things, special symbols and objects with unique meaning to you and your love in celebration of your sacred bond.

Create your traditions as a couple in the way that reflects your creativity and imagination, your life and how you live it. My husband brought me a scarf from every place that he traveled to. When I opened my closet I could see his love and our years together and our connection throughout his journeys in the world. When he was gone, I wrapped myself in the colors of a scarf and let myself miss him, long for him, and looked forward with anticipation to reuniting with him.

When he was with me, he still mailed postcards to me from our home to our home because I was the one who picked up the mail. When I came home and went to the mailbox, he had often sent me a postcard with a love note, a little poem he had written for me that let me know I was special to him and that he thought about me and was passionately attracted to me.

A Feast of Love

I offered him food to show how much I loved him because he loved me. I prepared the food he enjoyed with great intention and served it to him carefully with love, on special plates that had meaning to us. He enjoyed things that are colorful and pleasing to the eye, so I paid careful attention to please him with my choices of food, glasses, cups, and linens. I chose things that had an interesting character.

I showed him I was thinking about him in how I attended to his body. I said *Here, eat this soup my love, it will give you the best health and you will live 100 more years so that I can love you for a long, long time.* I put herbs, fresh vegetables, and greens on a beautiful plate and I said *My love, I have put 10 things here that will make you strong and healthy. They already taste very good, and I also put my love into this dish and I give it to you with my whole heart and body.* These special things had meaning to us.

Magical Words and Creation

Words are spells, so that's why I imagine we call learning words *spelling*. We need to be very careful about the magic of words and use them with our love. What we say matters and calls upon the magical forces of life. The thoughts we give each other, every touch, every word we speak is either building or tearing down our love, withholding intimacy or generating it.

Be very careful with what you think about your partner because they will feel it. Give loving intentions to each other at a spiritual level, as well as the physical. When you make love, really do *make love*; think about what you are making and speak what you are making with the magic of words.

When I had a difficult test at school as a girl, my mother would give me a little bit of chocolate and say with great love in her eyes, *This magical chocolate I give to you with my heart and wishes will help you get an A.* Was that chocolate magical? Perhaps, or it could have been her faith in me and the care she took in taking care of me that powered me successfully through that test to return with the A she had helped me receive.

Why not add magic to everything? When my daughter coughs, I tie a scarf around her neck, kiss her, and say: *This magic scarf will make your throat better.* Everything is for good luck and for love. When my husband traveled, I blessed him to be safe and return to me, and he swore he could feel the difference.

There are rituals from traditional marriage ceremonies that we tend to be drawn to subconsciously, whether we think about the symbols or not. Why do women love to have fresh plants and flowers around? To create the energy of nature in a temple of love. Why do men give women flowers? They are honoring the Goddess in their woman.

The exchange of rings matters because it creates an unending circle—a symbol of love returning and renewing. Give each other rings for special occasions—so as to create and recreate love. Sharing music you love and creating lots of playlists you can enjoy together fills your home and bedroom with the muse of love in ways that will serve you well.

Make your bedroom unique. Your bedroom must be free of electronics—there may be no television and computer in your bedroom if you want to sleep deeply and make love to your partner in a magical place. There must be a balance of space in a bedroom between the space taken up by the man and the woman. She can't have clutter and craft projects everywhere, and he can't dominate with exercise equipment. The bedroom is just for sleeping and lovemaking and absolutely nothing else. No office in the bedroom. If you have to, put your home office in your garage or on a porch or absolutely anywhere else, but never in the bedroom. Cell phones are put to rest in another room for the night.

The bedroom is your holy place. The cleanest and most beautiful place in your home. If you want to know what you are currently emphasizing in your life, do this. Walk through your living space. If sex and love are important, this needs to be seen in how your bedroom looks, feels, and functions.

Have a thriving plant or small tree in your bedroom. Take turns watering and fertilizing it so that it holds the magical intention that as the plant grows, your love will grow too. But don't be so superstitious that if the plant happens to die, you think the relationship is over! Just enjoy the ritual of attention placed on something together that you can grow and have as a symbol of your love becoming stronger, putting down deep roots, and reflecting the care you are putting into your relationship.

Feed each other berries and grapes in bed and say in a ritual way what you are feeding each other. I am taking care of you. I am feeding you in ways that will make you successful and strong and happy. It's fun and sexy and it bonds people to each other. Speak the magic of the words, *I will love you and feed you when you are old, I love and feed you now, and it gives you strength, power, and joy, my love.*

Seven

Looking With Healing Eyes

Peace Is Worth More Than Money

I was fourteen. I was in love. The boy's name was Viktor. I wrote letters to Viktor but did not send them. I stored the letters in a drawer, the only place I could call mine. My brother and I shared a small walk-through living room. There were two beds and one table in the living room; one drawer in that table was mine. When I was seven, I had a very special place to store my most prized possessions. I dug a small hole in the ground in a beautiful park right next to our apartment building. In that hole I stored beads and pieces of colored broken glass. Now at fourteen, I had stopped digging holes in the ground; I had my very own drawer.

One day I came home from school and walked into the living room. I saw my mom standing next to the table. In her hands she was holding the letters, *my* letters. I screamed and snatched the letters out of her hands. "How could you…" I ran outside; I ran to the park. I should have buried them. I was devastated at the violation of my privacy. The hole in the ground would have been a much better place to store my letters.

When I came home, my mom tried to talk to me. She was telling me how much she loved me, how much she wanted to be a part of my life, how she was worried about me. I said that I would never tell her anything about my life anymore. *Never.* The frightening, final word.

I was a difficult teenager. I struggled with my identity. At fourteen, I ran away from home. Not for long, but long enough to break my mother's heart. When I came back home, she had deep, dark circles under her eyes. I felt terrible. It took us some time to forgive each other, but I kept feeling the unspeakable sorrow somewhere deep in my heart.

Now I am a mother and I long to be close to my daughter. I walked into my daughter's bedroom and saw a piece of paper on the floor. I picked it up and read, "I love Andrew." *Love?* She was six years old! I was staring at the paper when my daughter ran into her bedroom. She snatched it out of my hands. "This is my room! *My* room!" I smiled and slowly walked out of my daughter's bedroom. I called my mom. I said, "Mom, I gave you so much pain when I was a teenager. I am so sorry." My mom didn't pause for even a second. "No," she said, "we didn't have many fights. You are a wonderful daughter, I am so lucky, and I love you so much."

"I love you too, mom, you know that, right?"

"You may tell me that more often," said my mom and smiled. I know she smiled because I heard it over the phone.

One of my friends lives with her in-laws in Russia. They fight every day. There is always something to fight about: how to raise her son, what to make for dinner, who will walk the dog, and so on. She feels literally drained of energy. Unfortunately, I know many families that fight every day. When one of their family members gets sick, they don't see the connection between the fights and the disease. But there is one. A very clear link.

Romanies believe that interacting with gadje (non-Romanies) depletes one's energy and that being with your family in a spirit of love and connection, with your taboro, replenishes it. Your home and your family should be your safe haven. Your energy (your spirit) gets recharged there so that you are ready to face the world the next morning with courage and strength. If you ask any Rom, anywhere in the world, what is the most important thing in life, the answer will always be the same: family. Romanies live with their parents and grandparents in the same apartment or house. Romanies respect their elders and love their children so much that it borders on worshiping. The great-grandmother has the most authority in the family. She is consulted when important decisions have to be made, has the final word, and no one dares to challenge it. Elders continue to play an important role in the family even after passing away as stories are shared and their influence continues.

Why this emphasis on family? I think it is a literal connection to the DNA and the bodies we inhabit and the ways in which they are linked. It is difficult to be in a physical body. We experience physical pain, emotional pain, and we struggle mentally and spiritually. But we all do the best we can. The struggles of life should unite us, not separate us. Gypsies are never alone. We never feel disconnected from our family and those who came before us. We live and travel through life in big families. It's a noisy, joyful, confusing place to be in the midst of a loving family. And what keeps things going is the ability to really care for each other and to forgive all of the large and small upsets that arise.

And so we arrive at one of the most important secrets to living a healthy and happy life. The ability to forgive others, and the ability to ask for forgiveness.

Forgive and Forget

Forgiveness creates a new beginning. In Romani culture, when someone is dying the word goes out through the network of family, friends, and colleagues, and even to people who barely know the person who is dying. The news passes from person to person. Everyone considers their connection to the dying person and looks deeply into their own soul. They ask, "Do I have any unfinished business with this person, a misunderstanding to be resolved, forgiveness to create with them?" It is an important and somber time. This is the final opportunity to face up to everything that has been done and what is left undone. It's the final opportunity to examine the hurts and insults, the bad treatment, the regrets, the things that if not forgiven will haunt the living after the person who is leaving has died.

If it is possible, people travel to be with the dying person and look into their eyes. They reach out and hold the hand of the dying person and make things right. This takes great courage, but a Gypsy knows it is worth it.

In the non-Gypsy culture around me when I see people fighting against death and denying it as if it can be avoided, I want to hold them close and whisper, "Die like a Romani. This is a precious time. Don't miss the magic." Birth and death are the sacred bookends to this miracle we call life. Birth is a time when everything slows down and becomes very quiet and a new life is welcomed with reverence. Death can be like that too. Slow down to let it be honored with reverence. Serve and help the people that are leaving this world. Receive the gift of forgiving and being forgiven by communicating wholeheartedly with the dying and you will have a longer and healthier life.

In our Romani culture we gather around the dying person to share stories. We laugh and cry. We sing and dance. Anything that needs to be said is said and there is a release that makes everything right. I love this ritual of my people.

To love life and to be free we need big doses of forgiveness and we don't need to wait for death to come calling to achieve this. There is an opportunity to live in the pure light of forgiveness every day if we are courageous enough to do it.

Ask for and receive forgiveness every day so that nothing is undone and unsaid. And always give forgiveness generously to keep your own health and well-being in balance and to be in harmony with the natural world around you.

Forgiveness to Make You Healthy

In big families, there is always someone and something you have to forgive. If you are lucky enough to have many friends, there will always be someone you have to forgive and be forgiven for as well. The act of forgiveness releases so much magical energy that it can be used for healing, making wishes come true, and creating magic in your life. It is very important to forgive everyone in your life, including *yourself*. And it is very important to do it EVERY DAY.

Begin with the past and clear it. What memories or wounds weigh you down and feel like a burden to carry? When you look closely you will see that this heaviness comes from needing to forgive and to be forgiven.

Think of the difference you feel when something is completely forgiven and you don't even remember what the fight was about. You feel like a clear running stream, a clean and sweet smelling breeze. Imagine if you could remain that free all the time because all was forgiven in your life. The power you will hold with that quality of soul cleanliness is incredible.

Recently I faced one of the hardest things a woman can cope with when, after my husband had been away on a few trips for business, I could sense something was very different. We loved each other. We were close and had a healthy relationship for fifteen years. I loved him very much and I knew he loved me. We were devoted parents to our daughter. Our home was a happy one. When he returned from these trips and I looked into his eyes I could see his pain. I asked what was going on with him and he knew not to deny my intuition. Women always know when something is going on with their men. And Gypsy women? He knew he had to tell me everything.

In a sad whisper he said, "I am in love with another woman." My response was to sob uncontrollably for two hours. This may be a difference in how I was trained as a Romani. Many women I know would shut down emotionally or would allow themselves to get very angry first. I know that anger is a mask for deeper emotion. I knew I was hurt and devastated and sad beyond the limits of what I thought I could endure. I let those emotions into my body without fighting them and they moved through me like a great wave or storm.

I will protect the privacy of my husband and the woman he fell in love with and not share more of the details, but what I can share is that their romantic connection had happened suddenly from a friendship they had established in childhood and they felt as if they were destined to be together in this way. My husband was also very sad and fully aware of the impact of his behavior. He didn't dishonor me by making it my fault or blaming something in our marriage. He accepted complete responsibility. He explained that he didn't seek out the relationship or plan it, and he expressed that he didn't want to do anything that would hurt me more than I would naturally be hurt. It had happened and now the reality of what was in front of us needed to be handled with as much love as we could gather.

At this point many adults would try to hide everything from their children—as if a child can't feel the energy going on in the home and sense the dynamic between their parents. Children pick up on everything. It's important not to over-share with children but to deny reality is to shield them from life and that's not possible.

I had been sobbing for hours when our daughter returned home from school, the house was full of my grief when she asked what was the matter. I told her the truth—without blaming her father, making him wrong, or putting my pain on her. I reported what had happened. Her father was in love with someone else. She started crying too. She went right to the sadness of the situation without anger or bitterness. She was brave enough to feel her pain and express it. We hugged on the couch and cried together. The three of us were in pain, two adults and a child, and it was a clean kind of pain because we were not adding additional wounds to each other.

I struggled for days to understand what had happened. I didn't make any big decisions yet. I let myself feel the confusion. My world was shattered and I needed to try and understand this with patience and compassion. I turned the tables in my imagination. What if I met someone, a sense of destiny was between us, and I suddenly loved this other man more deeply than my husband? What if I had to go through the pain my husband was experiencing? And how did this woman feel knowing the impact of their love on me and my daughter? What was happening in her world? How could my daughter make sense of this so that she could grow up to believe in marriage and love and also know the reality—that love can be a complex and unpredictable thing? That is a part of the magic of love—that it can come and go, or remain but shift like the tides of the ocean.

When I finally felt calm and in a position to look with healing eyes upon the situation we all faced, I called the woman my husband loved and asked her to share her experience with me. As I dialed her number my heart beat so hard I thought it would jump out of my chest. When she answered I listened to her voice and felt into her heart and mine. We would have a real conversation. She had loved him from childhood and now they were connected again. I had been with him for 15 years and now she felt it was her turn to experience that kind of love.

After our conversation I needed time alone to work through my hurt. I felt both love and hatred. Fear about my future arrived wave after wave and gripped my heart tightly. If I listened to those negative emotions and turned myself loose like a wounded wild animal, my family would be harmed. I needed to find my center. I did not rush it. I asked to be alone to read books and articles and personal stories shared on the Internet. Then I asked for advice and support from my community, my family, my friends, my taboro. I honored the complexity of what was happening and brought in an entire team of people to heal.

My compassion grew as I shared my pain and heard the pain of others. So many people had gone through this! So many of my brothers and sisters in the human family have known this particular kind of pain. People opened up to me as I opened up to them and I found that many were struggling in their relationships more than I had realized in the past. As I went through this experience I learned that to be of service to the healing of others I needed to understand this particular experience deeply. I found the gifts inside the pain.

How had so many of the marriages I knew in the Gypsy culture worked so well? How had arranged marriages with partners chosen carefully by each set of parents created long and healthy connections? There are divorces and there is heartbreak in Romani families. But there is often a deep respect for a life-long bond and a commitment to weather bad times that I'm sure makes a difference. There is an expectation that couples (and the community around them) will work hard and long to make a relationship successful and enduring.

Did I want to be married to my husband if it represented a sacrifice for him to be with me? What would it be like if he stayed with me out of guilt rather than something he chose with his whole heart? Did I want to be loved by a man in this fragmented kind of way or could I move on and be alone for a time to heal and then call in a man who would want only me?

I looked to my own actions. To make my life the best it could be, I made sure I was eating particularly well with the very best fresh food and dancing and exercising more than I had before so that my feelings would move in the world freely. I created new challenges in my life to keep myself fresh and engaged and happy to be alive. I got some new clothes that made me feel beautiful, made new friends, read more, helped other people, and found new sources of joy. I created a long list of things that made me happy and I did every single one of them. I proved to myself that my happiness depended only on me. I celebrated the truth that I am the source of my own joy. No one can make us unhappy if we are completely responsible for our own happiness.

Because of the pain of this experience, I was more sensitive and more in tune to others. I used that energy in my life and became more open, more curious, and I noticed people and things around me in more detail. I started using my imagination and intuition more. I became more alive and expressive and energetic. It was as if processing my pain gave my life a boost of rocket fuel and a greater capacity to love.

When you learn by experience that your happiness does not depend on anyone else, you have access to a deeper part of your own soul. You can be deeply confident in an unshakable and unstoppable way. You can be unpredictable, mysterious, and powerful when you let go of other people as the source of your happiness and power.

After some time had passed, I knew the right action to take. I told my husband that I was sure I wanted him to be free and happy. I couldn't control his actions but I could control mine and I could make sure that I put love and forgiveness at the heart of our family. By going through this together I became closer to my daughter and my extended family, my co-workers, and my communities, including my Roma taboro.

Rather than being a tragic experience, a scorned and wounded woman, a person full of complaint, our divorce sent me shooting high into the stratosphere. Men started to ask me out on sight and I got compliments from strangers—men, women, and children would come up and tell me how radiant I looked. I had fun every day. I glowed with happiness. I loved my life and I was complete and fulfilled on my own. This is the magic of forgiveness. I couldn't have experienced these breakthroughs if I was nursing my pain and holding grudges, judging, being a martyr, a victim, or finding fault with my ex-husband and his new love. Do you see? Our circumstance is only what is happening to us. We are the ones who make choices about what the story of our life means. We write the ending of each chapter of our life. We are the ones who set ourselves free!

Forgiveness Exercise

Take the time to slow down and make a list of the names and actions of the people who have hurt you throughout your life. The thoughts that come to you again and again will help you create this list. The stories you share about how you were harmed need to be rewritten so that you are not a victim in your life story. This is your work. If you can go through everyone and every action on that list and truly forgive them, you will live a longer and healthier life.

They have their experience of you. With an open heart you may be more able to see things from their experience. Often the people who carry the most pain are the ones who inflict it on others. See the story of your life from where you are now. Do you see how your difficult experiences have made you the person you are now? Do you see how "dark" times can bring the most light?

Now also think of the people who may have you on *their* list. What would they write about what you have done to them? What did you say that caused pain? How did the impact of your choices affect others? How may you have harmed others intentionally or unintentionally?

Imagine someone you may have hurt. Feel the impact of what you have done and said. Explore this from as many angles and per-spectives as you can. Take full responsibility for your actions. Don't defend or justify anything, just experience it from the perspective of the person you have hurt and stay with their experience in your own mind and heart. Do you want them to forgive you? Do you want to be free of that harmful tie to them and make it a light and loving connection? To make this exercise easier for you, I recommend a wonderful blend of essential oils called *Release* at the end of the book.

*   *   *

Sometimes it is important to reach out to people to have a conversa-tion and to generate forgiveness in person. Sometimes this cannot be done, but it can always be done at the level of your soul and theirs. You can write a letter and burn it and give the ashes to the air or bury the ashes in the ground and ask the Universe to deliver the message to their soul. You can talk to them in your mind and heart and send them messages of forgiveness and love every time you think of them.

If the person is close to you and in your life often it is best that you connect with them in person to seek and receive forgiveness while looking into their eyes. It's possible that you have hurt people and don't even know it. You might even try asking forgiveness of those close to you by asking them to share with you anything you've done that has hurt them. We often have these things hidden in our blind spot—out of sight just enough not to know the impact of our actions. By giving them permission to tell you, a new door is opened. You may be surprised to find out that most of the people you thought you didn't hurt will say, "I was so upset with you because…" and share something that you didn't know you had done. Every one of us has a different view of the world. Something that will make you laugh will make another person cry. Something said to one will roll off them like a warm summer rain and another will feel the same remark like a cold winter storm.

When you genuinely ask for forgiveness, the other person feels valued and appreciated. Try asking for forgiveness often and see how it feels to you. It is always worth the pain to open our heart wider because after this we feel so much more love and other people also seem kinder and more open. If you don't have the courage yet to speak your forgiveness or ask for it—try this. Do it in your mind, whisper it to yourself, speak it into the wind and ask the wind to blow your message into the ear of the person you can't face yet. Do this again and again so that your secret message is carried to the heart of the person you want to heal. You can build this muscle quietly in private and then over time be able to speak it aloud to others. As you forgive, so you will be forgiven.

Someday, when you are ready and have worked this new muscle of forgiveness, ask the Universe to forgive you for everything that comes to mind when you feel shame, sadness, and regret. When you do, the entire Universe will seem kinder and more open to you!

Gypsies understand the power of forgiveness and the importance of forgiving first and not waiting until the person who hurt you asks for forgiveness. This seems counter-intuitive to people, as if holding onto their wounds will create justice. "If I forgive first, before being asked, won't that let someone off the hook?" Yes it will. You! You will *stop* your own suffering. The most important benefit is that forgiveness frees you from pain no matter how wrong the person was in the way they treated you. If you don't forgive, you are the one who gets punished: punished by the way you relive the event again and again—wounding yourself many times over.

Imagine if the Roma held onto the hurts they have sustained for so long—the genocide, the persecution, the pogroms, the discrimination they have faced. What if that stopped us from singing and dancing? What if that kept us in the prison of sadness even though we are roaming free in the world?

Roma say, "Thunderclouds build upon thunderclouds as you recall grudges." Don't create your own misery by holding onto grudges or slipping into the use of bad language to describe yourself, others, and life. Don't label others with harsh words. Don't get stuck in the words you choose to describe the things that have happened to you. You already know how important the choice of words is to Gypsies. Positive words carry positive energy. Negative words carry negative energy. It is that simple. The spoken word is magic and we know it.

In Gypsy culture, if someone swears oaths of hatred even just around the dishes in the kitchen, these dishes will never be used again. They would either be thrown away, sold, or destroyed. Romani women go out of their way not to upset each other in the kitchen with the dishes in their hands because who wants to end up without any beautiful dishes? Every aspect of life is like that—keep yourself and your environment and your possessions in a space of love and forgiveness.

I had a client who came for a healing and fortune-telling session with me and she had terrible back pain. As our session went on to other subjects she never mentioned her back because she was focused on the suffering in her mind but it was clear to me that they were linked. Her mind was looking "backward" to the pain of very old relationships. She was full of pain about previous breakups and full of questions about her present relationship. She asked these questions in ways that were more linked to the past than to creating a different sort of future. She wasn't in her own life and experience in the moment of now. She was absolutely stubborn about not forgiving the people in her past. And she wanted me to look into the future—as if there was only one version of it. She wanted to see ahead in order to avoid any pain. Would the man she was with currently leave her? Would they be together in 20 years or would he abandon her? She was grasping at the future and holding onto the darkness of the past. Her back pain was one of the ways her body and soul were trying to communicate with her, but she wasn't listening. She had internalized painful experiences of the past at such a foundational level it was literally as if they had fused into her structure, her skeleton, and had become part of her. She was in misery because she was making herself miserable and I'm sure she was making her boyfriend miserable too and that if she kept this up he would eventually leave her as she feared he would—and was unintentionally causing to happen.

I did my best to help her heal. For thousands of years people have brought their problems to Gypsy fortune-tellers to ask for help in relationships, to heal broken hearts, to find true love, to restore their hope, to glimpse ahead. We do our best. But I can tell you one of the most magical things in the Universe is the forgiveness you can generate on your own. If you arrive in a relationship clean of the past you will create a loving future. Use that magic. It is within your reach every day.

I remember years ago complaining to my father that during the previous week the Universe seemed not to talk to me. I couldn't understand what was happening. All of a sudden, the Universe was silent. My father listened lovingly. As I complained to him my daughter walked in and asked me a simple question. I didn't answer. My father asked me why I didn't answer my daughter's question. I said, "During the past week, she was misbehaving a lot. I am punishing her by not talking to her."

My father started laughing so hard he nearly fell off the chair. I was very confused. He smiled at me, "Don't you understand?" No, I didn't understand anything. "When there is no harmony and forgiveness in your family, you can't be in harmony and at one with the Universe. And when you are not in harmony with the Universe, you don't hear the Universe talking to you even though it is, and this false sense of separation causes even more problems in your family." I saw what he meant instantly. What a great lesson!

Every day, before you go to bed, ask for forgiveness from every person you encountered during the day. And then forgive everyone who knowingly or unknowingly caused you pain. I guarantee that you will fall asleep with a smile on your face and the Universe will speak kindly to you in your dreams.

Problem: You feel lonely and isolated and need connection.
Solution: This is something that is not a common problem in Romani culture. Families are highly valued. Community is valued more than an individual. There are always people around to talk to and enjoy. Take personal responsibility for your isolation and loneliness because YOU have created it, and you alone can change your life the moment you reach out. Have you become out of touch with your family? Rebuild

close relationships with all the family members you can find. Forgive everyone! Get to know your neighbors. Make new friends at work. Join a club or organization connected to your passions. Join online groups and forums. Create a community of like-minded people. Organize pot-luck dinners and other events that gather people with food and music. We were never meant to live in isolation. Don't even try. Don't suffer alone thinking there is something wrong with you if isolation makes you feel terrible. Of course you are sad when you are lonely! The Universe designed you to be with others. Now get out there and connect!

Problem: You think you are not living with the right life partner.
Solution: Inquire more deeply into your own heart and actions first and don't look to your partner as the source of your happiness. Your partner is the person with whom you share the happiness you create in yourself and they will share the happiness they generate with you.

In traditional Romani culture, parents select the bride or the groom for their children. There is no dating, and marriages are arranged when children are teenagers. The divorce rate is very low. Why? In the modern world the divorce rate is very high although everyone mates easily, dates for a long time, and couples live together before marriage. You'd think that would be a recipe for stability and hap-piness but it isn't. It takes the reflection of others to see ourselves clearly, and love and support for creating a loving marriage comes from a community that is pulling for our success in relationship.

Many relationship breakups happen because we are looking for someone else to make us happy. If we search and find happiness inside ourselves, we start accepting our husbands or wives just the way they are and loving them just as they are and working on the marriage together. If something bothers us, we change ourselves instead of try-ing to change someone else. This way, we can learn, grow and change together, with love and respect for each other. This will bring a long and healthy marriage. Look inside first and then love outside yourself with an open heart and acceptance and you will experience lasting joy.

Living in the Passion of Red

When I advise people, and when I'm asked to share knowledge and work with people on specific aspects of their lives, I help them live in the passion of Red. Passion is something that can take practice because it requires courage. I help people find that courage.

When we put ourselves out in the world, we risk what people might think. Gypsies know it is important not to care what others think because of all we've been through. We've been despised and judged and misunderstood. If what others thought controlled our lives we'd be miserable all the time.

Changing your life for the better is something that has to be practiced. Part of the power to do this comes when you choose to live a bit louder. Can you take up more space? Can you place the color red around you to hold the energy of passion? Can you speak up and out? Can you dare be more open and bold? Try it.

In the Romani way we give a red ribbon to bring good luck when babies are born. We use red ribbons for protection throughout life. Red is not only beautiful but also holds sacred energy and life force. Use it.

Reclaiming the Word "Wish"

I blame Disney for watering down the meaning of the word "wish" so that it seems frivolous rather than absolutely powerful. It has become a small thing in our culture. But wishing on a star is a very big thing. Gypsy fairy tales are full of the word *wish* and it means something that carries great force and creative energy. To wish is to intend, to summon, to generate with magical power that is very real.

Modern science is proving the connection between all things, but Gypsies have always known that the energy that holds everything together is Divine and that all of us have access to that power as daughters and sons of the Universe.

Some people have lost their sense of how magical life really is. I will help you reclaim your full power to wish. Something that is very deeply connected to the soul, the soul's wish, is a spark of bright fire you want to ignite into a full and wild flame. When you know how to wish properly, the power of the Universe will align to create that reality.

In order for the spark to become a full fire it needs *fuel*. You cannot sit on the couch watching the lives of others on television and fill yourself with bad food, sleep poorly, and not express your love and passion and expect to generate a magical life. You will not.

Wishes are also not granted by someone knocking at your door and handing you the life you dream of—as if it arrives without effort. You must go into the magical wood for the kindling, and you must gather the firewood through your good work. You must go and create your wish and ask the Universe to help you.

You make your wish real by doing the active steps, struggling, meeting with failure, connecting with people who can help you, connecting with people who disappoint you, and still you must go on no matter what in order to make the wish come true.

When you take on life's challenges in this way the achievements are even more satisfying. When you stop being a lone wolf and trying to do it all yourself in isolation you will receive the joy of collaborating with your taboro! You'll do it together! The things that matter most are worth the struggle, worth the work, worth the effort and the faith it takes to create them.

Here is something Gypsies know very well. Your deepest wishes will show themselves to you when you are a child. The things you imagined, dreamed about, and longed for as a child will provide you with a map of what you are here to make of your life.

Go back to your childhood with the help of photographs and memories. Think back to your earliest happy times. What were your struggles? What delighted you? What were your favorite toys and activities? What were you curious about? Who were the people and animals and places that made you happy? Reconnect with that happy spirit from childhood and find the parts of you that are carefree, creative, and not conditioned by adults or society.

Forget the rules and the ideas you've accumulated over the years about what is possible. What adventurous and unrestricted part of you can dream big? What are your soul's *wishes*? You had them for a very specific reason. You were listening to a clear message about who you really are and why you were born. Now, slow down and stop the chatter and clutter of your mind and find that clear and clean sense of who you really are and begin to make every one of those wishes come true in the best way you can.

First make a list. Hide it if you have to so that you don't feel too exposed or vulnerable at first. Start gathering the resources to make those wishes come true. What do you need to know, who do you need to know? What actions do you need to take? Keep building this little treasure trove of wishes and dreams until this way of being feels solid to you and you can begin to share your wishes with others. Begin only with those you love and trust the most. Ask them to treat your wishes with tenderness and respect. Everyone knows you can't pick up a newborn baby and swing it around by the leg. Don't do this to your wishes and don't let anyone else treat your wishes roughly. Nurture them privately and kindly until they are sturdy enough and developed enough to withstand hearing the kind of criticism that could shut you down or pull you off course. By the time some people in your life hear about your plans, you'll need to be underway already and solid in your commitment to make your wishes come true no matter what. Then you can withstand things that aren't supportive.

When you are clear about what your wishes are, pray for them, invite support and protection around them, and hold onto your vision with everything you have so that your wishes don't fade away again. Keep your dreams brightly colored and powerful and strong. The Universe will respond because when you are doing the things that you are made to do, even though you will still face obstacles, you will persist and succeed because your desires—your powerful wishes—come from your deepest heart. You are here to fulfill your wishes.

Preparing for the End, Living Well Now

Illness and death are there for all of us, but many of us prefer that they arrive late in life and that when we leave we have enough time to say goodbye and forgive. A Gypsy will also pray not to linger around death so long that we suffer a great deal. This is what it means to have "a good death." To have this kind of death you must take great care of your body and mind so that they serve you for a long time—and then when it's time, you just go.

One of the best ways to invite this kind of magic into your life is to express gratitude to the Universe easily and often. The mind has enormous power with the body.

This power is well documented and I've seen it all my life. When the mind hears a misdiagnosis it can tell the body to become sick when it isn't and the body can shut down! When there is a terminal diagnosis, but the mind plays tricks and fears death, the end can sneak up on us and we don't get a chance to experience the end in a good way because we're in denial about it.

When there is an early warning about a disease that may be coming and the body is whispering to us through early symptoms, it's best to act to prevent, slow, or turn back illness by changing our lives, getting ahead of the healing, and taking great care of ourselves with gratitude for life.

We must be sophisticated about how we approach these things. To live long and be healthy and happy we must love the body we have and take care of it based on love, not fear.

I see people in this culture afraid of aging and dying. They eat out of fear, exercise out of fear, erase the lines on their faces by stretching and filling the lines out of fear, use medicines to mask the symptoms of what's going on underneath the surface rather than curing the dysfunction of the body—all out of fear. They are using their power, but in a dark way and it doesn't bring joy or a fulfilled life or good health.

A big part of my job is to help people see how powerful they are and to get them to use their power to create health and wholeness. It takes courage to be fully in your life working with your body—living an "embodied" life. Vitality takes effort and then it generates so much fantastic energy that you become a powerhouse!

When I met my husband he was suffering from kidney disease. It was thought that he wouldn't live long. We didn't buy a wedding ring at the time we fell in love because he didn't think he had long to live. We were celebrating life and love in the shadow of his possible death and that made our love even more precious to both of us. As soon as he let my Gypsy wisdom guide him and learn the proper diet, his health flourished.

For the years we were married I fed him fresh nutritious food. He loved the way I set up our home and how we used the magic of the Romani to enhance every area of our lives. Our love stayed fresh and alive for the time we had it, and our love ended with dignity and full release when it was time to move on. Often in the 15 years we were together people would assume we were newlyweds. Now that we are no longer together I wish him more of the kind of love we shared as he moves along in his journey in life. And I wish that kind of love for myself again too! I wish great love for my daughter when the time is right for that so she experiences that great joy. And I pray for my Romani family and for all my friends and my clients that each of us lives fully, in life and in good health.

When any of us have symptoms or receive a diagnosis we must take it very seriously. This is the time to use the very best of medical science to improve our health and well-being and to open our life to the contribution of the Universe and the miraculous healing that can be even deeper than a cure for illness.

It is even possible to get sick and die and be fully *healed*—from disappointments, to have received and given complete forgiveness, to love life up to the last breath. It is possible to make even the remaining limited time of a terminal diagnosis a time of celebration. When some people receive a terminal diagnosis they become angry, feel it isn't fair, lash out at others and create misery in their family in their final days. This means they have been denying the reality of death all along. We cannot be angry that we will die any more than we are angry that the sun rises in the morning. It is a normal and natural part of our life cycle. When we embrace this knowledge, every day becomes precious in good health or bad. This acceptance of death is part of the mystery and magic of life.

I have a client whose mother was known in their large family as a difficult person. She lived with some level of persistent complaint and seemed to feel like a victim most of the time. Then came a cancer diagnosis that became very serious. First she denied the reality that she would ever die and worked at her health and well-being as if she wouldn't die. But still, that was a positive change for her because it put her on the path of eating well. Next she read books that convinced her of the link between body and spirit and so she worked on forgiveness and love and enhancing her life. What happened? Her health improved so much that she often forgot she had cancer throughout her body. She felt good most of the time. Her life was extended a full decade and it was a higher quality of life than she had ever experienced before. But the best part of her life experience was the way she completed it by dying--whole and healed of many things. She pulled her family together and encouraged them to cooperate, to forgive, to be in each others' lives in a more authentic and loving way.

Years after her death the entire extended family points to the time they spent with this matriarch at the end of her life as an inspiration to live and die well. The positive impact on the entire family has continued. When she spent her final days in the hospital they gathered by her bedside to share family stories and to sing together. They laughed. They cried. They had fun. The doctors and nurses loved having this loud and joyful family in a hospital ward that was usually somber and sad. It was a memorable time of coming together and celebrating not just her life, but the lives of ancestors. They pulled together as a family and are still in close touch years later. This is a good death.

And then there are the clients who send death on its way for a nice long time. It is possible to cure an illness that is thought to be incurable. I have seen this happen many times. It is wonderful when this happens and the doctors scratch their heads in amazement. This isn't always possible, but when it happens we are grateful. I have seen so many medical miracles I could fill a book only with that alone. I have seen things for which there is no scientific explanation. The tumor that disappears from the scan and the surgery canceled because there's nothing to do but celebrate. I've seen the regeneration of nerves, the remarkable turnaround from organ failure to full health. We live in the world of magic.

My daughter was born very sick. Her illness was caused by a birth defect—she was born with three kidneys and two urine canals. We were told she had a severe infection and that we should prepare ourselves for her dying very soon. She went through two major surgeries—one right after she was born and another when she was ten months old. She had a resistant infection that was eating her skin. I gave her only fresh food and there were no such things as sugar, cereal or soda in our home. We ate fresh berries. We ate beautiful creations of nutrition and color. I taught my family that fresh mango pie was better than other sugary options.

Over the years the good life became contagious. My daughter lived and was perfectly healthy. My husband's health issues resolved. We didn't get the flu or colds when other families did. We lived well.

I showed them rather than told them. When faced with a buffet prepared by someone else, my family would gravitate naturally to what was the most nutritious food being offered, not because I told them to, but because they just knew what would make them feel good and be healthy.

No one likes to be scolded or bossed around. We all want to make personal choices without pressure. Encouragement and support are better. I had a private moment of motherly pride when my daughter became ill before an important party and said, "Mom. Make me better fast. Make me juice, add garlic to the salad, help me fix a hot bath with sea salt, and massage my feet with your magic oils!" Teenage daughters are dramatic. Of course, it all worked and she was in perfect health for the party. She will probably rebel in cycles like I did growing up. She may turn away from Romani ways at times, but I know she will always return to what it takes to live a balanced life connected to the natural world.

People ask us how we are so healthy. They are drawn to me to guide them. My healing practice came to me rather than me seeking it. "Please," people asked me, "What are your secrets?" I have to smile because I use so much Gypsy magic and their choice of the word is accurate -- these things really are very special secrets, but they can be shared with love at the right place and time.

As I give help I also receive it. When I'm faced with challenge in my life, my Roma family is there. Each time members of my family come to me for help, each time a client calls with a health issue, we work together to find the creative solution. As a big healing community we use the best medical science has to offer and the best use of Gypsy wisdom and we create magic.

One of the deepest secrets of health and wholeness is *community*—it is absolutely essential for health and healing. One day it will be part of medical insurance forms and hospital admittance procedures to check boxes about how supportive our friends and family are, if we have animal companions, how much time we spend outside with our feet on the ground, because that is a much more powerful influence on health than many other factors.

In the taboro at the first sign of trouble we jump in to ask, "What can I do to help?" We get creative. We ask for inspiration and support from the Universe. I pray and ask *please let me be open to receiving healing for this person, for my people.* When I get stuck and no answers come, I go outside in the most beautiful place I can and start writing without thinking and I continue until whatever I am writing starts to make sense to me. There are many secrets to connect with the wisdom of the Kingdom. I use all of them that I know and can discover.

Wealth of Many Kinds

"Rom has three horses and celebrates and is happy because he is rich, and the Count who is a rich man has three hundred horses and wants more." So who is really happy and who is really rich?

I love this Gypsy twist on a well-known phrase. "One who saves for a rainy day has a rainy life." Now that sounds counter intuitive but it's true. I know a family that has a "disaster fund" and a "disaster box" of paperwork and documents and they are so focused on disasters that they practically create them in the anticipation of them. There is nothing wrong with preparing and saving and thinking ahead about what might be needed in a crisis, but think of the difference in how it can be approached. They could have an "important papers" box and a "dream fund" instead, and their focus would be on the joy and gratitude they have to share, rather than on "disaster" they constantly anticipate as being right around the corner.

If you anticipate that the worst things will happen, you are postponing your life and replacing creativity and personal power with worry and anxiety. I worked with a client who at first thought he *couldn't afford* healthy and nutritious food because he imagined it was more expensive than other options that were cheaper. Have you ever had that thought as you reached for a cheap substitute to the freshly pressed nutritious juice after noticing the higher price? He pocketed the savings but was out of pocket much more by not being healthy and requiring prescription drugs and medical treatment for persistent complaints. I invited him to add up all the expenses he paid because of his persistent low-grade health. I invited him to immediately spend that money for healthy massages and great nutrition and rest.

Now think about this. We really are what we eat. We say that as if we understand it but very few do. The first medicine is the food we eat and it determines the quality of life. The greatest savings is to save our body from illness and disease. Spend more money on good food. Good health is worth *everything*!

We have a Romani story about the importance of treating yourself as if you are precious. "There was a man who had a shed full of bright, crispy, red apples but he wouldn't treat himself to the best one and would find the rotten apple and eat it. Every day he found the apple that had gone bad that day and ate it in order to save the best ones for later. During the year he ate 365 rotten apples instead of throwing out the first rotten apple and eating a fresh apple every day." The lesson is clear. Don't postpone life and save the best for later. Eat fresh food today. Use the good dishes now. Take the beautiful things down from the top shelf and put them on the counter. Do that fun, wonderful thing now. Fulfill your childhood dream now. Generate success around your wishes now. You have enough time. You have enough money. You have your life today, and that is precious.

In general, Gypsies don't save much money or food, and we don't accumulate things because we know that material things don't matter. We spend without guilt and our generosity is admired. We live in faith. Money is not worshipped. For so many years Gypsies have been poor and lived in poor conditions, but that hasn't defined our people because we see ourselves as bigger and better than our circumstances.

If a Gypsy family has money for a big house full of expensive things and rooms to get lost in, they would still want to be together in the kitchen and sleep outside under the stars. Money isn't valued more than people or the natural world. Not having money is nothing to be ashamed of, and for us it's easy come, and easy go, and who cares? We don't cling to money or worship it. Money is like air, or water, or food, it is there to nourish us, not to own us.

Everybody knows in their deepest heart that money can't buy happiness, but many people set up their lives as if it can and then are disappointed when they are not happy. Examine your own heart and how much you might believe that money will buy your happiness. A certain level of money is required to meet basic needs, but an increase in money beyond that simple and good life doesn't increase happiness. Celebrate and enjoy the necessities that are absolutely essential. Nutritious food on a table in a beautiful place where you are surrounded by family and friends is valuable. Your sense of purpose is your treasure. Good work to do is your wealth. A connection to the natural world is your fortune. That's what we really need and that's just about all we need.

Wishing and Creating

One day, I was house cleaning with the windows open, singing happily, and I found my journals from the time I lived in St. Petersburg, Russia. Here's what I had written years before: "I wish I could go to America. Life is so predictable here and so limited. I don't feel as if I can be myself. If I go the United States I will be thrown into a whirlpool of the exciting unknown. My life will be such an adventure. I wish for this opportunity." This was written years before an opportunity to go to the United States was even presented to me. I had completely forgotten that I had written it. Reading through my journal years later, I realized that most of the wishes that I had written down had also come true. Some things I wished for turned out even better than I had imagined. This is magic.

What do you wish for? Imagine anything, anything at all. I wanted to have more excitement in my life, to learn new things, to live a life I was very passionate about, a life that would make me really, truly happy. I wanted to find passion that would reach every part of my soul. I completely focused on that wish.

One night, I had a dream and it reminded me of a wish I had experienced as a child. I saw myself skating on ice. I was spinning and jumping, I was moving with grace and confidence. I felt as if I was flying! I was definitely flying in my soul.

I woke up feeling so happy! This seemed like a message from the Universe, so I decided to take a skating lesson and see if I would feel the same way in real life. Surprisingly, I did, although I was almost thirty at that time. When I began to ice skate I could barely skate forward but still it was fun. In just one year, I learned to skate forward and backward on ice, and to spin and even jump. Finally, after working hard and playing on the ice with all of my passion and love, I could jump high off the ice, rotate in the air and yes, feel like I was flying just as I had in my dream.

Figure skating became my passion, the real, true passion. I loved skating by myself, teaching others to skate, watching figure skating shows and competitions, reading skating magazines. I surrounded myself with the joy of skating.

I won my first gold medal in a competition and couldn't believe my wish had become a reality. I wished for the opportunity and made it real when I skated during the opening ceremonies of the 2002 Winter Olympic Games in Salt Lake City. I performed in the Theater on Ice. I was on TV, my photo was in newspapers and magazines. I was on top of the world!

Then, one day, I jumped up into the air but as I was landing, the blade of my left skate went straight into my right leg. I cut myself with my own blade. The wound bled a great deal and I was in a lot of pain. Injuries are very common among skaters, so I wasn't extremely upset. The wound wasn't deep and I thought, "In two weeks, I will skate again." But time passed and the pain did not go away. I went to see a physical therapist. He gave me a set of exercises, but as I exercised the pain kept increasing. I was now in more pain than when I had cut my leg. I saw an orthopedic specialist. He took some x-rays and said that all looked well to him and that the pain would just go away in some time. It didn't. I saw another doctor. He sent me for an MRI. The images didn't show that anything was wrong, yet I could not walk. I saw other doctors. One gave me a diagnosis that I couldn't pronounce or understand. Two of them said surgery was my only option to heal.

I couldn't skate. The source of my great happiness had disappeared and nothing replaced it. I went from being unhappy to being desperate, from desperate to depressed, from depressed to thinking my life was over. I wished for the pain to go away. Why wasn't my wish coming true this time?

Finally, I scheduled the surgery. The night before the surgery, I had a nightmare. I saw my foot being cut off. I woke up in sweat. The nightmare seemed very real. I needed to listen to the message of this dream carefully and get help in understanding what to do next.

Several hours before the surgery, I asked to speak with the doctor. I looked straight into his eyes and asked: "If I were your daughter, would you do this surgery on me today?" The doctor was silent for a moment and then said "No." I canceled the surgery and limped out. I was on a quest for answers.

Listening to the Wisdom of Pain

Months passed, but my leg did not get better. I stopped smiling. I reached the bottom of a very deep hole. It was so dark and it seemed there was no way out. And when I thought I could not suffer any longer and asked for help from the Universe with everything I had inside me, I had another dream. It was similar to what many people describe happens when their heart stops. I saw a very bright light. The beauty of this light was unspeakable. I slowly approached the light and became one with it. All of my senses reached their highest point and I was filled with love. The joy I felt did not compare to anything I had ever experienced. I became this light, and also kept my sense of self. I felt enormous peace. I was in a state of bliss and ecstasy. I woke up with tears of gratitude rolling down my cheeks.

I still felt the connection with this incredible light. To me, it meant the essence of the whole Universe. There was something about cutting my leg that I had experienced as if I was surrounded by a high wall that was keeping me from my beautiful life. I should have connected with the Universe sooner, but I had used logic to try to solve the problem on my own rather than remembering my Romani heart and soul. The door to the other side of my pain and limitation was open by feeling the connection with the whole Universe. I let go in trust and surrender. With the white light I welcomed all the pieces of my shattered soul back home. I listened to my pain and found my joy.

I realized that what happened to me was a great lesson. Figure skating wasn't supposed to be the sole focus of my life. It was supposed to be just a small part of it and I wasn't supposed to have my entire identity wrapped into the thing I was doing. I had stopped following my soul's purpose in the largest way and had focused only on skating as the source of my happiness. I had narrowed the whole world to just skating on the ice. I was missing the wonders and magic of the rest of the Universe!

Pain always provides an opportunity for growth. We only have to inquire deeply into what is behind the pain. We need to ask the right questions. The body is simply bringing messages through pain. Psychological pain is the same—the mind is showing us where we need to heal.

Pain is always an opportunity to stop and learn. It's a way our higher self communicates with us. We get too busy. Commitments keep us running. We desire things and chase after them. We seek a new relationship. We search for things that have less value than our connection to the Universe.

What happens when you finally get what you dreamed about? How long does it keep you happy? A year? A month? A minute? Or maybe you thought it would make you happy but it didn't. When we get sick or hurt it's just like a red traffic light: it tells us to stop. For some, pain is a reminder to stop desiring more of everything. For others, pain is a reminder to stop going in the same direction and move onto another path.

Use your pain to get you out of being stuck in a pattern that does not serve you any more. In my persistent pain I changed my wish from simply being on the ice and framed it differently. I now wanted to find happiness through interacting with the larger Universe. I wanted to learn the language the Universe speaks. I wished to see more of the interaction between us and the Universe and that gift was granted to me through my painful time. I learned my lesson. I have the joy of not feeling separate from the Universe. My pain has opened up new realities to me.

Healing Eyes and Blessings

The concept of the "evil eye" (Basavi Jakh) and of curses is well known in Romani and Russian cultures. Their opposites – *healing eyes* and *blessings* -- are less familiar to most people, but obviously are much more important. Here is how the evil eye works: a woman (in our teaching I have never heard of men possessing either evil or healing eyes but I don't deny its possibility) simply looks at her victim. She concentrates her feeling of hatred on the victim and especially on the victim's eyes. This very negative energy is multiplied if a woman curses the victim either silently (less harm) or out loud (more harm). The destructive energy has the potential to "stick" to the victim and can cause all kinds of harm, sickness, and ill fortune if this person is not protected. Gypsy women have used the power of the evil eye and the curse throughout history to retaliate when they have been violated, raped, humiliated, and persecuted. My sisters who use their power wisely only use a curse in extreme circumstances and in advance such as preventing a rape by creating a field of protective energy around themselves and stopping an attack. Revenge is something that causes more pain. Protection is always called for and is needed in rare circumstances. There are other protections that are more common.

A common teaching of the Romani people is that newborn babies are especially susceptible to negative energies created by the evil eye. Russian Romani even limit the number of people who are allowed to see the baby until he or she turns one month old. Only the closest family members are allowed to be with the baby or to look into its eyes. Even pictures of the baby would not be taken or shared during that time. It is believed that the evil eye can curse even by looking at the picture of a person. Gypsies also isolate the mother and the newborn for several weeks after birth to keep them protected when they are both so open and vulnerable.

In contrast, in the United States, I've seen newborn babies taken to a busy shopping malls and being looked at and spoken to and touched by many people--strangers. It is true that many people will look at the baby with admiration and love, but others may look with jealousy, judgment, or even anger if the baby starts to cry. A newborn is far too delicate for this kind of treatment. That is why they require special protection.

The *healing eye* works in a similar way, producing the opposite results of the evil eye. A woman looks at an injured or suffering person with the most love she can possibly feel. She concentrates her feelings of love on the wounded person and especially on the injured person's eyes. This very positive energy is multiplied if a woman blesses the injured person either silently (less healing power) or out loud (more healing power). The beneficial energy "sticks" to the injured person and will create healing and attract good luck.

Romani also understand that when we look into the eyes of someone who is in love with us and when we are in love with them, we feel enormous uplifting energy. This energy of love can create miracles.

Russians say "Eyes are the mirrors of the soul. Everything one is feeling inside opens up to others through the eyes." Consciously concentrating this energy can bring a lot of destruction or healing depending on one's intent. This is true even for blind people. I know of several blind people who have the ability to see the future and who are famous healers. My own spiritual quest has led me to develop the ability to see with my eyes closed. I cultivate this gift and am grateful for it.

Not only do we send energy through the eyes, we also receive energy through the eyes. People who spend regular time outdoors in the sunlight tend to sleep better at night and have more energy because when the sun enters the eyes, the hormone melatonin is produced and it is this hormone that is responsible for regulating sleep. This is the scientific explanation. By now you can feel the deeper truth. When you connect with the Kingdom you are held by the power of the Universe in health and wholeness.

Looking at beautiful pieces of art or places in nature also creates a very positive energy in our bodies. How thoughtfully do you work with the energy of your own eyes? Do you choose what you see carefully? Develop your power of intention when you are looking at anyone, even strangers. If you catch yourself focusing your eyes on someone with any degree of harshness, train yourself to catch this negative energy and transform it to love and compassion. Look with kind eyes on all.

Never give anyone the evil eye. Ever. Do not send bad intentions to people through your speaking or through your gaze. Do not let words of gossip leave your lips. There is a reason that every major world religion prohibits gossip and makes it clear that it is very harmful. Gossip may seem harmless, a way to blow off steam, or pass along information as if it is a fun pastime. But if you sow these damaging and dark seeds through your eyes and your voice, you will reap a harvest of unkindness. Talking about someone to share loving concern is very different from gossip, and the soul knows the difference. Your body experiences the difference. Your eyes see the difference. Do not look at someone with ugly thoughts in your mind. Do not look at someone and be jealous of what they have or speak in ways that tear them down. Thinking or speaking judgmental thoughts is poison for you and the person you are speaking about.

If you notice that you are looking at someone and thinking dark and unkind thoughts 1) immediately look away, 2) close your eyes to shift your energy, 3) concentrate on softening your eyes by thinking a kinder thought, 4) look upon them again, now with kind eyes, and 5) both bless them and ask for forgiveness in your heart so that you have fully shifted the evil eye into a loving eye. Once you have had to catch yourself this way and take these steps to clean up the energetic mess you almost made, you will remember the next time you think to look unkindly.

In time and with practice you will stop this detrimental behavior, and your life, mood, and health will elevate. Others will also be drawn to you because of your kindness and the positive energy you hold. I have a client who mastered this so well after only a few months of practice that total strangers approach her in public places and ask, "What is it about you that is so different from most people?"

What should you do to deflect the evil eye coming at you from others—either intentionally or just out of sloppiness and lack of awareness? Surround yourself with anything that is positive as your first defense. Think a very happy thought, or think about a loving or beautiful thing as quickly as you can because beauty and love are stronger than anything negative. The evil eye will be deflected successfully by love and kindness. Carrying special charms will protect you from the evil eye as well, because charms do have energy. When you respect and cultivate positive energy and remember it whenever you see the charm, hold it, and always have it with you, it will offer real protection.

A charm is an object that is filled again and again with positive energy. For Gypsies a charm may be gold and silver coins or symbolic amulets, something beautiful to wear and keep close. What you think you need as a charm will depend on the intensity of the evil eye coming in your direction.

If you treat others with more love and respect, you will naturally receive less negative energy coming toward you and will amplify love moving towards you.

I've been asked about the kind of random anger that is sometimes directed from a person who is mentally unstable ranting on the street. This is very different from the anger coming from a person who is psychologically well, who knows you, and has the conscious intention of hurting you. The person who is mentally unwell can be easily deflected by loving eyes and compassion and blessing them in your mind or softly speaking aloud.

This is rare, but real curses are sometimes used by some Gypsies, who in turn risk being cursed themselves as a result of using curses on others. I won't tell you about any of those curses because I don't want them added to the world. I would only ever use a curse as a last resort if someone was being attacked, to protect children, or to prevent rape. Curses should only be used as protection in very extreme circumstances.

The healing eye, on the other hand, is something to use every day with everyone you meet. It is the most beautiful thing you can share, and it creates so much positive power! You can physically feel it when someone is looking at you with absolute and unconditional love in their eyes. Sages, saints, and great teachers often possess this power. People will stand in line for hours to be seen by a guru of any faith who has mastered looking with loving eyes, knowing that it is worth it to receive this blessing. You may feel your heart open and your hair stand on end when someone looks at you like this. No touch is needed for this to be healing—just the look is enough.

You may have special healing gifts that can make your healing eye even stronger, but everyone can choose to look at people with kindness, love and acceptance. This makes a very big difference in their own life as well as the life of the person who is being loved through the eyes.

I've worked with so many people over the years that I believe that every person has some level of this magical ability. It doesn't take special training, because it is your birthright as a human being. The energy of love is absolutely universal and everyone can release this energy, increase it, deepen it. What you send out into the world comes back to you. This is a fundamental law of nature.

I have seen many times that even one use of the healing eye will generate positive benefit, sometimes in unexpected ways. Miracles happen. The unexpected unfolds. You will find that giving the healing eye doesn't drain you of your own energy, and in fact, it fills you up. Love can only uplift, fill, and increase joy and health. Love does not drain or deplete. If you are always tired, you are not experiencing enough of the energy of love in your life—the love of humanity, love of animals, love of nature, love of everything around you.

Loving and Being Loved

The people who come home drained from work do not *love* their work or the people with whom they work. If you love your work, the people you work with, the place where you work, the time you spend doing it—all of that love will feed you and others. Children know this very well. If they are playing a game and doing something they really love, they don't want to be torn away from it. You can't get them to stop. They glow and skip and laugh and if you look in their eyes you will see healing energy and joy. We can learn so much from children.

There is a beautiful Gypsy blessing: "Let your children be healthy and happy and joyful and live for a hundred years!" Speak those words with love and kind eyes and you will create magic. The word in Gypsy culture is very important. We know that words are magic spells and that the choice of words matters. Never speak ugliness. And it's better to be silent than to say random words that don't have any value or power. I notice that often times people just chatter thoughtlessly and say things out of habit without paying attention to what they are saying. What they don't realize is that the words they speak are creating their lives and relationships. Their words will be reflected in their environment and what comes back to them.

Know that what you say becomes real. Guard the magic of your spoken words. Don't use your words thoughtlessly. Use them to create good things and to generate healing.

Problem: You sense that someone is looking at you with jealousy or hostility.
Solution: First of all, avoid feeling fear, jealousy, and hostility yourself. Like attracts like. Second, surround yourself with beautiful, sparkling light at the bottom, at the top, to your left, to your right, at the back, and in front of you. Imagine you are being protected by

a shield of loving energy. No negative energy can penetrate your energy if you create it well.

Problem: Your energy level drops after spending time with certain people.

Solution: Your body is trying to tell you something, so do your best to avoid these people. If this is not possible, use your healing eyes on them. Imagine sending them the most positive, loving energy you can create. What you send is what you will receive. As soon as you have created a higher vibration in your life, people who are a lower frequency will naturally gravitate to be with people who match their frequency, and the new level of energy you have created will be matched by new people coming into your life who are aligned with your new energy.

Problem: You suspect you may have been cursed by someone who is sending you unkind energy and you sense you are feeling the impact.

Solution: If possible, travel to a beach and swim in the ocean to receive the cleansing of salt water from the earth. If this is not possible, rub sea salts into your skin and rinse with a cold shower while praying for them and releasing the curse. You cannot be harmed if you protect and clear your energies.

In the Palm of Your Hand

A friend of mine is blessed to have a mother who has healing eyes and can see inside someone's body. She sees the disease and she can help the healing process by using her eyes and voice. She's been known to completely heal terminal cancer patients. I wanted to meet her and learn from her. My friend's mother, Svetlana, lives in Odessa, Ukraine so it took some effort to be with her.

It took me twenty-four hours to get to Odessa. I was completely exhausted when I got there. Svetlana was free to teach me in a few days and I decided to explore the city while I waited to see her. I went to the downtown market, which was also a gathering place for local artists. I struggled to adjust to the time change. I was tired and sleepy. Nothing special caught my attention until I saw a booth with beautiful crystals. An elderly gentleman who had a great energy offered to help me choose one when I told him how beautiful his crystals were. "Please give me your hand." He looked thoughtfully at the lines on my palm. As he held my hand gently in his, something extraordinary happened. It felt as if he transferred the energy of joy to me, giving me a big dose of happiness. I knew how to read palms, but I wanted to learn how to do this transference of joyful energy and asked if he could teach me. He said "Not yet. I see that first you have to gather some information about the Language of the Universe and share it with others. You see this line, when it reaches the one in front of it, you can be a healer who offers deep health and well-being. Here, this crystal will help you."

The palm holds the map of destiny of a person, but the life journey is still full of many choices. The future is created with the Universe as your partner and it is there to read in your palm as well. To Gypsies, reading palms is simple. It's like boiling water or trading a horse. Gypsy women are in touch with their intuition and speak clearly, and so this is easy to do. Your life is in your hands and your life also has elements that have been predetermined. There are aspects of your life that are destiny or fate, and that shows up in your palm. But what you do with what you have, how you experience your life, and what you make of it are yours to live freely. Life needs to be full of surprises. It is interesting to peek at the future and to know something of your destiny and fate, but you are still responsible to make your life and your future. To live fully requires you to live in the present. If you knew everything in advance, it would not be satisfying or bring you joy because you'd be ahead of yourself, fantasizing and connecting with the future, and you'd miss the present. But if you don't have any sense of what's possible, you could miss the chance to let your destiny call you and pull you toward it. You see, it's a paradox. The future is both knowable and not knowable.

To live a healthy and joyful life you can't be too much in the past or the future. They are both important--but you've got to focus on the present. Palmistry is a useful tool every once in a while, but it must be done rarely, with respect, and with the understanding that things in the present can have an impact that will change the future that has been glimpsed but is not promised.

Reading the palm is reading the future, and Gypsies usually don't want to know the future because we want to live in the present moment right now. I know that I create my future. I am in charge. I'm going to create it in any way I want. I don't need advice about how to create it. On the other hand (sorry about that pun but it's perfect so I have to use it), there is no use to glimpsing too much ahead because that eliminates the joy of living and the surprise and delight of seeing it fulfilled. Gypsy culture is rich with feelings. They are not bottled up or restricted. Feelings are not covered up. We do not pretend we are not angry when we are, and we don't pretend we are not sad when we are sad. All feelings are expressed fully. One of the first things I noticed when I came to America was that people are very polite, even falsely polite, even when they are burning hot inside. When something is really bothering them, they will tell an untruth when asked how they are and answer, "I am fine." Even positive emotions are suppressed. When I'm happy at work, I literally jump with happiness. When something wonderful is happening, I smile ear to ear, I clap my hands with delight.

It is important to live authentically. Try this: the very next time someone asks you how you are doing, stop, think about it, share from your heart, and watch how the magic of life unfolds. "I'm struggling today. Thank you for asking." People are full of love, even strangers. We want to know about our brothers and sisters. If something really bad has happened and you share it, you will find support and caring. Your emotions are not something to be ashamed of, they are what make us alive.

So many people are numb and walking around like ghosts because they don't allow themselves to feel. If something bad happens that makes them feel hurt, the first thing they do is cover it up, suppress it as much as possible with distractions that make things worse. If you don't fully express your emotions, you are more likely to reach for unhealthy fats and sugars, numb yourself with television, drugs, or alcohol.

Watch children who are full of vibrant life force -- they do not contain or suppress their emotions. They let it all out and move through their emotions without becoming stuck. They are sad and then something makes them laugh. They are frightened and when that passes they are courageous and happily engaged. They clap with joy. They laugh so hard they fall down. They are not stopping life force, they are dancing with it. You can do this too and it won't be odd or unwelcome. It will delight people to see you flow with what you feel. Don't be afraid of this.

People often appear to be flat, as if they have same mood all throughout the day, but that's impossible! We are energetic beings at any time of the day, and it is natural to feel better or worse, happier or sadder. If you look the same, act the same from the beginning of the day to the end, you are managing too much. You must express your emotions to be fully alive. Feel and express.

Be authentic. Don't smile when you don't feel it. Learn to smile honestly. Don't paste a false smile on your face and leave it there, but let it come and go naturally. Big smile, small smile. No smile. Bigger smile. You are not wearing a mask, your face is your communication with the world and the world will read its impact on your face when you are authentic. Do what feels right to you.

Birds of a Feather

Birds of a feather flock together, and like attracts like. This happens everywhere you go. Those who complain get together in little circles of complaint and life appears awful to them. People who smile easily draw those who also smile to them. On social media it has been proven that if someone who posts an unsmiling photo connects with a group where smiling photos are posted, they will soon update their photo with a smiling one. We are who we choose to spend time with, so be conscious of your choices and use each of them to create the magical life that calls you.

There were many people waiting in line to talk to the gentleman who sold crystals in Odessa that magical day I followed my dreams and intuition, so I bought the crystal, thanked him, and left the market feeling enormous joy, wanting to skip instead of walking.

Finally, after my preparations, I met Svetlana. Even when I talked to her over the phone, I was mesmerized by her voice. Now, this feeling multiplied. Her eyes seemed to radiate incredible light. She spoke very softly, but each word was powerful. When I was in the same room with Svetlana, even silence seemed to have a meaning, and the room was overflowing with luminous energy. When Svetlana spoke, I had a feeling that now everything would be all right in my life and that the whole world is a beautiful place. It simply couldn't be any other way.

We talked about this and that and then Svetlana said "Let me show you one book you must know." She showed me a book by well-known Russian ophthalmologist Dr. Muldashev.

The book was called *In Search of City of Gods*. She said "This book is meant for you, you will find it fascinating and it will change your life in an unusual and exciting way. You will find this book in the store called Terra Incognita (the Unknown Land)." She then named two streets to help me find the place. The store was to be located on the intersection. I wrote down the names of the streets, thanked Svetlana and reluctantly said goodbye. I was sad to leave. It was as if I traveled to a magic land and now it was time to go back to reality.

The next day, I decided to find the bookstore Terra Incognita. I easily found the intersection but ... there was no store there. I walked around the neighborhood, up and down the streets. No luck. After circling around for twenty minutes, I found another bookstore where I asked if someone knew where "Terra Incognita" was located. They knew and gave me the address. I wrote it down on a piece of paper and hurried back. I found the building but it was a library! There was no store there. I was so tired from walking back and forth that I decided it was enough for the day. I slowly went back to the bus station. I wasn't searching any more; I was just looking down at the sidewalk. I glanced at the windows of one of the basements and ... saw the sign "Terra Incognita." I froze. It was there all the time; somehow I missed it several times! I went in. There were three different books by Dr. Muldashev and I bought all of them because I felt the pull to learn what he taught. Dr. Muldashev is the only doctor in the world who has successfully performed combined eye transplantation (cornea and retina). He returns the ability to see to blind people, to the ones who other doctors say, "have no hope." He has done what others claim is "medically impossible."

I still had some time in Odessa and I spent it reading the books and taking in my surroundings. Dr. Muldashev wrote about his trip to Tibet in search of the gate to Shambala, or the City of Gods, where heaven meets earth. Dr. Muldashev was not only a gifted ophthalmologist, he also understood the spiritual significance of eyes. He wrote about the secrets of the eyes depicted on sacred temples in Nepal. His adventures led him to the discovery of the differences between live and dead water and that led to the creation of solution he later used in his unique combined eye transplantations.

Eyes. Water. Medical miracles. The search for heaven on earth. I didn't have time to finish reading all of the books in Odessa. I came back home and kept reading. Dr. Muldashev shared that there is a place in Tibet where what looks like mountains are not actually mountains. This is what's left from a city built by previous civilizations. Some structures were built in a way that distorts the space around them and even time. He shared pictures and drawings of the structures that he found.

I sat at my table, reading page after page and going on the journey with him. Once in a while I would stop and think about the mystic powers of previous civilizations. There was a road atlas of the United States lying on my table. On the cover, there was a picture of the Delicate Arch in Utah, and I felt drawn to it as if discovering it for the first time. It looked so perfect that I wondered in a moment of creative dreaming and imagining if it also was built by previous civilizations.

As I stretched my left arm to grab the map, I glanced down at my hand. There is a distinctive red birthmark on my left hand. I was born with it and many people have asked me what it is, but I didn't know. Now, however, it looked like an arch to me now and something clicked newly. Suddenly, I realized that it looked just like the Delicate Arch. The shape and even the color were the same! I experienced it as a sign. I had to go to Moab now and see the Delicate Arch. I opened the map of Utah and started checking the names of big rocks on the map. There were more surprises. I found a rock that was called "The Looking Glass Rock." Dr. Muldashev had found a similar rock in

Tibet. It was called "The Mirror of Time." I was astonished by the similarities in the name and shape. Dr. Muldashev had experienced the rock as a thinking being that had consciousness. If one were to stand in front of the rock, one would get access into the parallel universe! If you have a connection to a special rock, one day you will know how magical it is to engage with nature in this way. Until it has happened keep your mind open. A tree may connect back with you when you take the time to connect with it. Being silent and peaceful on a big rock may create a connection with that rock.

I went to a bookstore and bought several books about Utah. I picked the ones that had big, colorful pictures and began looking through page after page with one thought in mind: What if these rocks have been shaped by beings from previous civilizations? I was allowing my childlike curiosity to pull me toward things I found interesting and fun. I looked for symmetry, pyramids, castles, similarities to human sculptures, animal sculptures, bells, windows, eyes.

I turned a page and delighted in a picture of a rock in Goblin Valley State Park. The rock had astonishing similarity to monuments located on Easter Island in Chile. I opened Dr. Muldashev's book and compared the pictures of the rocks from Utah to the monuments on Easter Island. My next step was to find Easter Island on the map of the World. This tiny island was located in the Southern hemisphere. I moved my finger up following the meridian and … I couldn't believe my eyes: my finger pointed at the Eastern part of Utah, the exact location of the Goblin Valley State Park. Both monuments were located on the same meridian! What fun! Did it mean anything? All I knew was it was much more interesting than numbing out in front of the television to have this project of following impulses and clues.

If the thought of seeing the Delicate Arch gave me a feeling of joy, the pictures from the Goblin Valley gave me chills. Although my little "discovery" was interesting, I found that I did not want to visit the Goblin Valley, just like I never wanted to watch movies I found scary, and something about those rocks struck me as scary in that moment. But I was powerfully drawn to the arch as if it was calling me.

I already knew that a physical shape distorts the space in a certain way. The shape of an object has a specific purpose. A bell has a certain shape and it produces certain vibrations. I wondered if even when the bell is silent, it could produce a higher vibration through its unique shape. A shape may produce feelings and thoughts of a certain nature. When I looked at the Delicate Arch, I felt elated and joyful.

The next day, I came to work and was called to a meeting in the office of a big boss. I'd never been in his office before, so I began looking around, glancing at the pictures on the walls. One of them immediately captured my attention. It was a picture of a mountain that looked exactly like a man's head. The similarity was striking! After the meeting, I asked the boss where the picture had been taken. He had taken the photo in Bryce Canyon in Utah. He later gave me a copy of the picture. I decided to go to Bryce Canyon one day but first – Moab. What kind of magical surprises were waiting for me in Moab? I couldn't wait to get to Moab and see what would unfold before my eyes.

Sacred Stones

As I was driving to Moab, the feeling that I was approaching a land I would find sacred was getting stronger and stronger. The shapes of the mountains were the most unusual. Gypsies believe mountains have a very powerful spirit. Some are inhabited by Little People (similar to how other cultures describe fairies or gnomes). Mountains that have unusual shapes are considered sacred. I saw a rock that looked so much like a sheep; it definitely appeared more like a sculpture built by human beings than like a rock changed by wind and time.

My first stop was Looking Glass Rock. I was surprised to find that there were absolutely no tourists around the rock. It was shaped similar to the "Mirrors of Time" in Tibet described by Dr. Muldashev and other authors who had a chance to see a glimpse of the parallel universe. It was shaped like an amphitheater, with a small "window" on one of its sides. The Rock was so symmetrical, so perfectly shaped that I had a strong feeling it may have been created by human beings from previous civilizations, and I let my imagination run from geological time to create a more fanciful explanation. I am sure thousands of people passed by this Rock and didn't feel anything unusual. But to me, it was absolutely magical, and I soaked up the energy of the place for a very long time.

I walked to the center of the amphitheater and, with my heart pounding very fast, I made a wish. Here is what I wished for: During the time of my birthday, I wanted to learn something that would change my life in an unusual and unpredicted way. I didn't know what it would be. I wanted the Universe to surprise me. After that, I snapped several pictures of Looking Glass Rock and drove to Arches National Park.

The short hike to the Delicate Arch seemed like eternity to me. Why was I born with this unusual birthmark? What would I learn when I saw the Delicate Arch? A turn, another turn, and finally I saw it. The view was spectacular. It was so much more than I imagined. I walked straight to the Arch and touched it. Not many tourists dared to walk straight to the Arch – there was an abyss surrounding it. I wasn't afraid at all. I knew I was protected. The tourists were probably amused looking at me walking around the Arch. I stopped and hugged it, I talked to it, froze in silence for minutes to feel the energy of the arch. What happened at the Arch could only be described as an amazing energy exchange between me and the sacred land and stone. We connected. Once we completed our conversation I went on to the Needle Overlook. I listened to my heart and I had a feeling as if I had finally come home. I took off my shoes and walked barefoot on the warm rocks. The view was breathtaking. It was so quiet and peaceful. I didn't want to leave this place. I was literally on top of the world! The rocks were alive; I already knew I could communicate with them. I return to this place in my mind and relive this moment over and over. I remember every detail, the temperature of the rocks, the color, the freshness of the air, the feeling of being weightless. I was one with the nature around me and in me, and it was with me. I memorized how it felt, so that I could recreate it later and make it last.

In Gypsy shamanic tradition, mountains and big rocks are connected to the Lower, Middle, and Upper worlds at the same time because part of the rock is buried in the ground, part of it is at our eye level, and part of it touches the sky. These are places and connections to savor and hold with reverence. If every human on the planet felt this connection to nature even just once, we would all know how important it is to care for the Earth -- our home -- as she cares for us. There are secrets whispered in natural landscapes that only our spirit can hear.

What can you do to increase the health and harmony of your life? Connect consciously with nature in every situation. Even if you live in a small city apartment, you can bring a stone home and place it where you need support. Do you want to anchor your health? Place it in the kitchen. Your restful sleep? In the bedroom. Your career? In the home office space. Use your intuition and listen to what opens up for you.

I place stones in my backyard -- lots of stones. I feel their protection and support. I feel their strength and power. I invite you to pick up stones from places you are drawn to and connect your home and work space to places that bring you joy. Surround yourself with memories and energies of beautiful places in nature so that each time you touch or look at your surroundings, your mind and spirit are connected to that place.

Problem: You don't feel enough support in your life.
Solution: Find the biggest rock in your area or travel to the mountains to connect with a stone that calls you. Touch the rock with your bare hands or sit on the mountainside and close your eyes. Imagine the strength and the power of the rock or the mountain transferring to your body. Feel the empowerment and support energizing you. Before you leave that place, find a small rock and bring it to your home or office. Any time you need extra support, simply hold that rock in your hand.

Look at the maps or globes that call you visually and think about the places that have called you in the past. Have you seen and experienced the places that pull you? What journey can you go on to open your life to new magic? When we travel, it is easier to let go of hurt from the past and create new levels of healing. The newness of the place signals to our brain that we are ready for new things. Many great stories of transformation begin when someone listens to the call to go somewhere and answers it. Where are the places that call you? Will you answer?

Your Wish is My Command!

After coming back home from Moab, I could hardly wait until my birthday. Would my magical wish come true? What would it be?

Finally, the day came. In the morning, I went to work as usual. I love my work because it bridges medical science and the new discoveries that I know will be more magical. I began reviewing studies that involved human subjects. We would learn more about what was possible as we explored the borders of the known and took steps into the unknown. One of the studies was about those who were very sensitive to light, noise and touch. As I read the study, I made one discovery after another. When I was a child, I always asked my family members to turn off the lights and to turn down the TV when I was going to sleep. They would reply, "But there is just a little strip of light down the corridor and we can barely hear the TV." Still, it was too bright and too loud for me. Everyone thought I was "too sensitive" to the light, too sensitive to the noise, to being hot or cold, to the way clothes touched my skin, to strong smells. I craved order, peace, and beauty more than others seemed to, and some members of my family found it annoying. They asked me to stop being ridiculous and to make an effort to change. I tried my best – and couldn't. Sometimes I suffered and wondered why I was born that way. And here I was on my birthday reading this groundbreaking study.

While learning about people with similar sensitivities, I suddenly realized that I could turn my "sensitivity" into a deeper gift. If all my five senses were very strong, my sixth sense, or intuition, must also be very strong. Thinking back, I remembered when I would call my friend and she would tell me "I was just about to pick up the phone to call you." Or I would give a present and hear "This is exactly what I wanted and wished for, how did you know?"

It was time for a birthday gift. I wanted to learn how to develop extrasensory abilities and signed up for a workshop. Students were paired up with each other at random. I had to put my hands on top of the other person's palms, close my eyes, and imagine I was entering the other person's energy field. The first time I did that, I saw a string of beads. I mean, I SAW. Just like seeing with my eyes open, I could describe the beads exactly. When I was done, I opened my eyes and was astonished to see that the woman I was paired with was crying. She said that when she was a little girl, she could see beautiful strings of beads, things that were invisible to others. She would play with them and they made her very happy, as if she could touch the magic. No one knew about this. But as she grew up she lost her ability to see them. She said that the fact that I saw a string of beads in her energy field made her remember this feeling of happiness and realize that if the strings of beads are still in her energy field, she could go back to that state of happiness any time she wished. And maybe, one day, she could see her strings of beads again. She thanked me, as if I had given her permission to be happy again.

Then, another older woman asked me to do a "reading" for her. I put my hands on her palms, closed my eyes and imagined entering her energy field. I saw the letter "B" which suddenly turned into a bird and flew high in the sky. Then I saw her swimming in the ocean. The bird was flying above her. I finished describing what I saw and opened my eyes. The older woman was crying too! What was going on? She said that she recently lost her husband Bill, and that she often thought of his soul turning into a bird flying above her. She had a ticket to go to Hawaii but she was afraid of the water and was not planning to swim in the ocean. What I saw made her feel that her husband was watching over her and that it was safe for her to go into the water.

Then, the leader of the workshop asked us to do the readings with the intention of seeing the guardian angels of helpful presences that were with the other person. I did my reading for a woman named Doreen. As soon as I put my hands on hers and closed my eyes, I saw two trees. I was a bit disappointed. I expected to see the angels. I told Doreen what I saw. She replied that a few days ago someone had given her two trees as a gift. She didn't know where to plant them and was thinking about giving them to someone else. She now realized that she received these two trees for a reason. She decided to plant them in front of her house and they would be her guardian spirits. "At least I did not make her cry," I thought.

Doreen asked me if she could try to see what my guardian angel looked like. I agreed. This time, she closed her eyes and put her hands on mine. In a few moments –she was sobbing! She didn't say a word, so I was getting uncomfortable. What did she see that made her sob? Doreen opened her eyes and said that she saw incredible light around me; the light was so strong and so beautiful that she got overwhelmed with the feeling of bliss. It was too much for her and she could not stay with this light any longer: the feeling was too strong. Her description reminded me of my own celestial vision. Her seeing this was such a discovery for me! I didn't know that the celestial light was still around me this long after my vision. It meant I could go back to it any time I wished.

I also remembered that day that my soul's purpose was to be a bridge between the visible and invisible parts of the Universe and to bring magic into everyday life for myself, my family, my taboro, and for many others. As I completed the book you hold in your hands, I remembered the magical gentleman in Odessa, the one who told me to wait until one of the lines on my hand reached another one before I began my healing work with many other people. I've seen clients over the years and transformed many lives, and now the line on my palm he pointed to is completely connected and I have collected enough knowledge about the language of the Universe to heal many, many more. The next step of my destiny includes you, dear reader. Your wish is my command.

A Few Extra Senses

Any time I have followed the vision of a journey to a new place, I connect with my soul and my purpose. As soon as I had returned from Moab, my extrasensory abilities blossomed. The interaction with the sacred land that called me created an exchange with the Earth, and this benefitted my life. I felt more creative and more capable. Everyone I know who listens to the call of their places and new adventures reaps a harvest of new energy, ideas, and benefits.

I invited more magic into my life and the Universe responded. I began having unusual experiences more and more often. One day at work I saw a picture of an ocean on my screen saver and suddenly, I heard the sound of the waves crashing. It was loud and it was real! It was as if I was sitting on the beach listening to the ocean. It was an incredible and very powerful experience!

Driving my car in silence, I suddenly began to hear a violin playing. The music was so beautiful that I didn't want it to stop. I heard the violin again at other times, once during a meditation journey with drums. I look forward to hearing it again and learning about the source of the music when, and if, this is revealed to me. The Universe sometimes takes its time.

The more I opened up my skills, the more opportunities to learn showed up in my life. I studied with masters, read extensively, and learned whatever called to me. I explored numerology and it helped me to find out that I could trust myself instead of constantly searching for some guru from which to learn. My intuition also a new, higher level with everything I learned. One day curled up comfortably on a couch reading, I set the book aside to rest and looked at the ceiling. I studied the paint patterns on the ceiling and let my mind play: this one looked like a horse, this one – like a cloud...Then, I began reading the next chapter. It was about looking at the ceiling searching for patterns! The chapter described exactly what I was doing. It was as if I had skipped few minutes into the future and "read" the chapter ahead in my mind.

I began having fun playing with my intuition. I would surprise people waiting in lobbies for an elevator. It didn't matter how many elevators there were: two or eight. I always knew which elevator was going to open 100% of the time. So, I would stand next to the elevator that I knew would open up first. It was a delightful game.

For fun in the past I had made bets with my husband about teams in the basketball playoffs. I was always right, but I realized that I could only see few minutes into the future, although I sensed that with practice, I could see further and further into the future.

Unfortunately, an event happened that stopped my intuition for a time because it frightened me to take on the responsibility for what I saw, and I was confused about how much of what happened around me was my responsibility.

I was driving to work early in the morning. The Sun had just risen and was shining straight into my eyes. It was hard to see the road, even through my sunglasses. I passed a woman standing next to the crosswalk with an orange flag. Her job was to walk into the middle of the road and stop the cars, so that children could safely cross the street on their way to school. Suddenly, I had a thought: "A car is going to hit her." I kept driving, struggling in my head about whether or not I should turn around and warn her because I wasn't sure it was real, a vision or warning, or a dark thought that had flashed in my mind. Finally, I turned my car and drove back to her intersection. It was too late. She was dead. Her body was in the middle of the road, next to the car that hit her. I was devastated. I didn't know if I could have prevented this accident. I didn't know what would have happened if I had talked to her. What did it all mean? For some time it hurt so much that I shut down my intuition. If I saw things, did that make me responsible to change them? I asked to understand and I was given great teachers and lessons that trained me to be more sophisticated.

When what I see is very easy and beautiful, I glimpse amazing things and my heart beats faster. I am excited. If I glimpse the future and see something devastating and painful, I may want to shut down, but now I know that if a vision has been given to me it has been given to me for a reason—not that I'm responsible for everything about that vision, just that I do what I'm given to do. I say what I'm prompted to say. I act as instructed and I trust that all will be well, even when it doesn't seem to be so.

Life includes pain and pleasure. Life always brings something we think of as good and something we think of as bad, but this is all based on our interpretation. We find it easy to live when we are experiencing things we find to be good, and when something we think is bad happens to us, we create that meaning and suffer. When I saw what was going to happen and it happened, I felt the pain of that and part of the lesson for me was that people die in accidents every day and that this is the way things work sometimes. There is no possible way to prevent accidents from occurring. Loving life even though accidents happen is the work of being human.

What is the definition of your fate? What is supposed to happen will happen if that is the way it is. The person who can see the future can't change it and does not have the right to interfere with someone else's destiny unless it is their destiny to do so. I give confirmation when something good is going to happen because I know I have been invited by the Universe to do so. If someone is really sick and I glimpse into the future and see them absolutely healthy and well, I tell them. This knowledge gives them the strength and courage to overcome their illness. If I see a healthy person who is healthy and happy now and glimpse into future and see the person alone, sick, and so forth, do I have the right to tell them this? I would say no because what if my words are the catalyst for them to give up now? If they thought that was the only thing that could happen in their future, they might start living their future of sickness now. Perhaps there are many good things to come before this difficult time. If I tell them what I see for their future now, they may start suffering right away rather than living fully and appreciating life—which might also alter their destiny.

And if someone is on their way to a miserable future, they can always interrupt that with bold, courageous action. I sat outside with a friend under the colorful tent of a vegan café, providing in-depth advice about establishing a diet of mostly raw foods. I was passionate. I was probably a bit loud in my excitement, waving my arms, encouraging my friend to choose foods that are full of life. Suddenly a man from the table next to us stood up and approached me. He handed me a piece of paper with his name and phone number, said that he overheard the conversation and was curious to talk to me. Then he left. I wondered about this man who appeared to be shy and perhaps even a bit disturbed. I called. We met at the same café a few days later and he shared about his divorce, his struggles to find his spirituality, the panic attacks he was suffering from often, and a persistent desire to kill himself. He asked for help. I shared the importance of the right foods—the ones that make us feel good physically and emotionally as well as spiritually. I gave him things to do to connect immediately with nature and people. He was a very good student. He implemented my advice starting that very day, and his transformation was spectacular. He runs into my office now, without an appointment, because his intuition is extraordinary about when I will be there. He is happy, healthy, and has a big smile on his face. "Milana, you won't believe the life I live now…" And he shares his stories. Sometimes he reminds me of the way he used to be, and we have fun with the contrasts of the two completely different people— the one he was before and the one he is now. He is well in his body, mind, and spirit. He got his life back and created it to be much better than it had ever been, all because he was willing to experiment with everything I had to teach.

What can we make of our lives? What are we thinking about and with what sort of energy? We are in a dance with our destiny, and so we might as well enjoy every moment of life and soak up everything we can. Living is our great gift. We can find many creative ways to unwrap that gift.

Eight

FINDING THE TURTLE ISLAND

Tears Won't Please, the Smile Wins

Gypsies know that happiness comes from when we laugh more than when we cry. Laughter banishes sadness. When I was twenty-three, I moved from St. Petersburg, Russia to Columbia, Missouri. I rented a tiny room. It was a space the size of a walk-in closet. This rented room was in a big house with a porch, and I would go outside every night and look at the stars. I moved in at the end of the summer and the nights were so warm! It was as warm during the night as it was during the day, and this was very new to me. Growing up in Russia, where the night meant cold even during the hottest summer, I was delighted by the discovery that it could be warm during the night! The crickets sang their beautiful songs, the stars were so bright that I thought I could touch them, and it seemed that when I was on that front porch alone every night, I traveled into a land of fairy tales!

My time in Columbia was amazing. There was something very unusual going on. Strangers would smile at me on the streets. I looked at them, puzzled. You see, strangers do not smile at each other in Russia. The first time a stranger smiled to me on the street, I turned my head back to confirm that there was no one behind me. No, there wasn't anybody, that smile was for *me*. At first when people smiled at me, I thought perhaps they knew me or thought I was someone they knew. In Russia, there were certain unwritten rules about smiling.

Rule number one: Children could not smile in class at school. (I got several F's just for smiling in class). Smiling was considered the same as daydreaming, which meant not being serious and not paying attention.

Rule number two: You could not smile when your picture was taken for documents. The official version of us that was known to the government had no sense of humor and did not smile.

Rule number three: You could not smile at strangers. Life in Russia was about survival. Each day was a struggle. When you frequently don't have heating and hot water even during the winter, when you have to freeze at a bus stop for up to an hour and then ride in a bus so crowded that people are squeezing you from your right, your left, your front, and your back, and when you have to stand in lines for hours to get food (or any other necessities) – smiling is the last thing on your mind.

So here I was, in the United States, among students who smiled during class, among strangers who smiled at me everywhere I went, in a photo studio where the photographer would make faces in order to make me smile to take my picture.

I held out for a month or so but finally I gave in. I took a deep breath … and began smiling at strangers. All the smiles that were bottled up during my life in Russia were released. Out, out to the world, free at last my smiles flew. I felt so free that I smiled at everyone! More and more people would casually tell me, "You have a beautiful smile!" or ask me "Why are you always smiling?" How could I explain to them that I had to catch up for not smiling for such a long time? My smile was like an explosion, coming from the bottom of my heart. My happiness was complete.

I decided to conduct an experiment. I would establish the first day of a powerful new habit. For one day I would smile all day long no matter what. And not just a false smile; I promised the Universe I would smile from my heart with a wide and authentic smile all day. I decided that the more difficult life became on that day, the wider and more real my smile would become in response. The morning went fine, until my little daughter had a tantrum because she could not decide what to wear. I was not going to give up my smile, so I put a sock on my hand and pretended it was a puppet. This puppet had a funny voice and was the "king of all clothes." It helped my daughter select the right clothes and we had a great time! When we were in the car I asked my daughter to tell me, "Smile," if she caught me not smiling.

But my biggest challenge was to keep smiling when I was passing by strangers on my way to the café for lunch. Would they smile back? I had never smiled to strangers in Russia and didn't know what to expect. I told myself that Gypsies are joyful because we are children of the Sun. The Sun shines on everyone. I told myself to be like the Sun and share my warmth with everyone around me! I kept smiling and noticed that most of the strangers smiled back. During that day, I learned a lot about myself and my fears and limitations. I saw the world in a different way too. After that experiment, I began smiling more and more often, until it became so natural to me that it began being difficult NOT to smile. Smiling has become my default.

After a while, everyone began saying how happy I seemed. One day an older custodian at work, who was always gloomy and silent, came to clean my office. I would usually drop a short, "Hello" to him, but this time I smiled wide and asked him how he was doing. You know, not the usual "Hi, how are you?" but "How are you doing today?" with a genuine interest to find out if something was bothering him. He lit up! He had almost no teeth but his smile was beautiful! He told me that he liked to clean my office because any time he came in, I was always smiling.

I began to love making other people smile. Gypsies admire those who have a sharp wit, who are able to improvise and joke around. Romanies highly value humor. You don't have to be a comedian to make other people smile. An honest and open smile is contagious. But being silly once in a while certainly helps to lighten people up. I had a coworker who was full of surprise and delight. She was very competent and professional, but then every once in a while she would hide under the desk and jump out to surprise us and laugh. Everybody loved her. She left me a sticky note with a smiley face when I was away from my office. Those simple little notes would instantly change my mood into a happy one.

The little things are often the sweetest. One day, my seven year-old daughter was in a very bad mood. Nothing would please her. Bad moods are contagious, and I didn't want to get it. So, I decided to try an experiment. I told my daughter that I'd like to "make" a smile on her face. She replied that it is not possible to "make" a smile. I asked her if I could at least try and she agreed. We walked towards a mirror and I told my daughter NOT to smile until I told her that I was done. She looked in the mirror as I used my fingers to gently pull her right cheek up. Then, I pretended to pull an invisible string to wrap it around her ear, so that the corner of her mouth would be "held up." I did the same with her left cheek. She was laughing by the time I was done.

Smiling is the first and greatest tool for creating happiness. The most important thing you can do for yourself right now is to smile! In a matter of seconds, the smile will warm up your heart and the hearts of others. Even if you are not "in the mood" for smiling, there are many exercises that can help you make it a practice.

THE SMILING EXERCISE

Challenge yourself: try not to become angry, no matter what happens in a day. Try to remain in a state of happiness. Create an atmosphere of kindness and keep the inner light shining. You can begin this practice as if you are playing a game to see if you can do it, and soon it will become such a habit that joy will be an almost constant state.

When my daughter is sad, I ask her to show me what a sad person looks like. I tell her to go ahead and exaggerate. Show me a very, very sad face. Then I ask her to show me what an angry person looks like. A scared person? A surprised one? And finally I ask her to show me what a happy person looks like.

This way, she trains her subconscious to be able to change from being sad to being happy by following her body language. You thought your facial expression reflects your mood? On the contrary, your mood follows your face. Change your facial expression and your life will follow.

Now my daughter changes her mood from a bad one into a good one on her own. When she is very upset and angry, she goes into her room, closes the door, and in a few moments re-appears with a smile on her face. Now all she needs to put herself right is a chance to read a few paragraphs of a good book, or a quiet moment to think and reset her mood.

I keep one of my favorite books next to my computer in the office at all times. Often I don't even have to open it. Glancing at it is enough to remind me how easy it is to switch to a happy mood.

Often, the Universe sends me little "smile reminders" or "smile messengers." During a particularly hard day at work, I decided to take a break and go to the cafeteria. I stepped into the elevator and pushed the button. A woman stepped in just before the doors closed. Usually, I would greet strangers in the elevator, but this time I had no strength to even be polite. I just stared at the closed doors. She said, "Just smile." I turned my head, confused, not knowing how to respond ... and smiled! Immediately, the world around me changed. It seemed as if a cork had popped out of a bottle and out flowed champagne. My eyes lit up. Someone else had shared their happiness, and now I had it too. The elevator stopped, the doors opened. The woman said, "There you go," and left the elevator. I passed on the gift by inviting others to smile.

Another day, I was walking to work and a man on a bike passed me. He stopped, turned around, and said, "Smile!" Weeks later, I was checking out of a hotel in New York. It was five o'clock in the morning, and I had slept only four hours. A poster on the door of the elevator said, "SMILE." For me, magic happens with elevators.

Be like a Gypsy and don't change to fit in with your surroundings unless they are lifting you up to an even higher level. Never become less than who you are because you are worried you will stand out. Your life is yours, so be unique!

SMILING ALL DAY EXERCISE

I challenge you to repeat my "smiling all day" experiment. Notice when you stop smiling. Is it when someone cuts you off in traffic? When you feel lonely? What makes your smile return? Are you smiling when you are alone in the room, all by yourself? What is your usual facial expression when no one can see you? It is very important to feel good when you are by yourself. When tranquility reigns in your soul, there is peace and harmony in your inner world. When you feel great alone, people will feel great around you. Otherwise, no matter how hard you try to project a positive mood, people will still feel that there is chaos in your soul and will subsequently avoid you. If there is genuine joy in your soul, people will be drawn to you to warm up near your soul's flame.

Smiles not only change the way we feel, they also change the way we think. If you have a problem that appears to have no solution, smile in silence for ten minutes, not thinking about anything. Then re-visit the problem and see what happens. New thoughts will arise from a joyful place.

Fitness for Your Emotions

Everyone knows at least a few exercises for the body, and so I have created a fitness exercise for emotions to build up your emotional health and wellness. Choose a positive emotion. Try joy as an example. Now pretend you feel joy. If you were joyful, what would your face look like? What about your posture? What would you say? Practice, or just play as if you had all the joy in the world, and then FEEL it. The more you do it, the more this emotion will become a constant part of you. This builds your emotional freedom and range.

* * *

How can you be emotionally fit with anger? Expressing appropriate anger is important so that it doesn't become buried in the body. One of the best ways to express intense anger is through songs and dancing. Gypsies could not express anger at non-Gypsies because if the taboro was at the edge of a village and anger was openly expressed, a policeman could turn everything inside out, burn things, and treat everyone disrespectfully. How could they express anger? By singing and dancing wildly, which gave permission to process anger and sadness well. You can do this too. Turn up the music and let go of the intense emotions inside. Give them a way to leave you and be taken to the heavens.

Your Magical Day

To create your perfect life, start with creating a perfect day. As soon as you wake up, smile. Make it a habit to smile even before you open your eyes. Let your very first thought be one of gratitude, and as your feet hit the floor say, "Thank you!" Send love and light to all people on Earth. Wish for all people to be healthy and happy. Then send your wish for the day to the Universe. During the day, smile each time you see yourself in the mirror. Smile each time you take a sip of water. At the end of the day, fall asleep with a smile. You will be surprised how everything in your life will just fall into place when you embrace the entire Universe.

Dr. Norbekov, a famous Russian healer, wrote a moving story in his book *Experience of a Fool or the Key to Regaining Your Sight*. He met an old man who used to have Parkinson's disease. The old man was now fully recovered and absolutely healthy. Dr. Norbekov asked how that possibly could have happened, and the old man replied that he went to a temple in the mountains. He didn't pay much attention to the story the man told him, but the next year he met four old men who used to have incurable diseases and now were absolutely healthy. It turned out they also had visited the temple. This time, Dr. Norbekov listened carefully to their stories. The temple was called the Temple of Fire Worshipers. The healings were so miraculous that Dr. Norbekov decided to spend as much time as he could at the temple and see everything with his own eyes.

When he got to the temple, he was greeted by the monks. "We are asking you not to sin in our temple. The one who sins will help us carry the water." The sin was to be gloomy! It turned out he had to smile all the time.

Dr. Norbekov got caught not smiling during the first day. The punishment was to walk four miles down a steep hill and then carry sixteen liters of water back. As soon as he came back, a monk approached him and said, "Please bring more water. When you were walking up, you were not smiling." So, Dr. Norbekov went down the hill and up the hill again and again, carrying the heavy load and smiling with an unnaturally wide smile. The only way he could accomplish that was by keeping his spine very straight.

A week passed and no visitor was caught without a smile. Everyone's posture had also changed for the better. At the end of his forty day visit, everyone, including himself, had changed. The changes were so drastic that every visitor asked the monks to come down and stay with them in the village. But the monks did not let anyone stay for long, and they did not leave. They wanted to create as much peace, happiness, and health as they could, and this was best done at the temple.

When Dr. Norbekov returned to his town, he was shocked by the gloomy faces he saw everywhere. He got a group of people together and taught them to walk with a straight back and a wide smile. This alone helped many of his patients get rid of their diseases and live a happy life. Do you believe that straight posture and a joyful smile will make a difference in your life? Let's try it and see.

Problem: You feel indifferent and lethargic.

Solution: Stand in front of a mirror, stand up straight, and make silly faces. Create ten different smiling faces. Open your eyes really wide. Smile with only half of your face. Start laughing in different ways: very quietly, very loudly, like a baby, like a man or a woman. Laugh so hard that your belly and entire body start shaking. End with looking with as much love as you can into your own eyes.

In a kingdom far, far away, nine hundred miles from here, ten thousand miles from there, there lived a king. He had a daughter, a beautiful princess. She was smart and she was kind. Only one thing troubled her father: she never smiled and she never laughed. Nothing brought her joy, nothing made her happy. The king tried everything he could think of: he invited the best fools from his kingdom and even from other kingdoms. They entertained the princess all day long with jokes and comedic acts. But the princess sat on her throne, as sad as a dark cloud, staring at the floor, not smiling even a little bit. And for that people called her Princess Unsmiling. So the king sent his messengers to remote areas of his kingdom. The one who will make my daughter smile, the one who will make my daughter laugh, will get her hand in marriage and the whole kingdom on top of that.

The messengers galloped throughout the kingdom, visiting every corner, and visiting a Gypsy camp as well. One of Roma said, "I will ride my horse to the Capitol; I will make Princess Unsmiling laugh." When he arrived at the castle, he left his horse at the gate and waited for his turn. Finally, he appeared in front of the princess and said, "I know, Your Highness, how to make you smile, but I can't do it here, in the castle. Come with me to my taboro; this is where I will make you smile. And if I do not make you smile, chop my head off my shoulders." The princess pondered a bit and, to the great surprise of everyone in the ballroom, agreed. "Servants, gather my things," she said, "I am going with this Gypsy." The king objected, but the princess had her way. The servants filled several big chests with everything for the road, but the Gypsy didn't agree, saying, "No, Your Highness, if you come with me, you come without servants and without chests full of things." The princess agreed, perhaps because he was so handsome. They walked out of the house and approached the gate. Unfortunately, someone had stolen the Gypsy's horse. Oh well, he couldn't do anything about that and so they walked barefoot on the beautiful ground, noticing the animals around them. One hour, two hours, three hours passed. By nightfall they entered the forest. The Gypsy said, "We'll stay here for the night and keep walking tomorrow."

"What will I be sleeping upon?" asked the princess.

The Gypsy took off his jacket and placed it on the ground. The princess sighed but couldn't do anything about it; she was exhausted. The Gypsy woke her just before the sunrise as the fresh air smelled of the magic of the earth and sky. "Wake up, You Highness, let's greet the Sun!"

"I can't, I won't," said the princess. "Open your eyes for just a moment," insisted the Gypsy. The princess opened her eyes and at this very moment the Sun appeared above the tree-tops. The princess couldn't take her eyes off it because it was so beautiful. She looked in awe and a smile barely touched her lips.

So they kept going, picking delicious berries along the way, listening to the birds, watching the butterflies flutter in the Sun's rays. At last, they came to the Gypsy camp. The princess and the Gypsy sat next to the fire, ate some mushroom soup, listened to Gypsy songs, and watched the Gypsy dances. Later, the princess fell asleep in a tent, with a smile touching her lips.

A day passed and then another. The king got worried about his daughter. He jumped on his horse and took off, along with his servants, to find the princess. When they arrived at the Gypsy camp, what did they see? The Princess dancing around the fire, smiling and laughing.

"You, Gypsy, what an enchanter," said the king. "Come with the princess to the castle. We'll have a wedding and the kingdom is yours."

"No," said the Gypsy, "we'll have the wedding right here. And the kingdom: does one need a kingdom if one has the entire world?"

The Gypsy in the story was good friends with Baxt. Baxt is a very important concept in Romani culture. It means good luck. People who know how to magnetize good luck to themselves are very happy. Baxt has a spirit, and it selects people it wants to visit. Baxt can stay for one hour or for one day. Baxt can get to like the person and stay with her for a lifetime. Baxt likes to hang out around children, and, most of all, it likes smiles, laughter, kindness, and celebration. It has a personality just like you do. Wouldn't you like to stay longer in a clean, comfy, friendly house full of vibrant colors, joyful music, and laughter? Baxt would too.

The Harder Your Life the Bigger Your Dreams

In days gone by, a taboro gathered around the fire and Roma took turns telling stories.

"Listen, I know of a place in the forest where wishes come true. You don't even have to utter a word. Yes, that's right, simply imagine what you'd like to come true, one and only one wish. Close your eyes and imagine your wish has already been granted. And there! You have your wish. Where is this place? Well, I will tell you. Wait until the first lonely star appears in the sky.

Walk towards that star. Walk until you reach a small forest meadow, a glade. Only take an offering with you. Place the offering in the center of the glade, sit down, and close your eyes. Imagine that the wish you have in mind already came true. Then open your eyes and say, "Thank you, Veshitko Dad."

Hearing these words, one of Roma jumped to his feet and said, "I will go find this glade." Everyone looked at the sky. There it was, the first lonely star. The timing was perfect. "Fair wind to your back!" said everyone. So the Rom walked towards the lonely star. An hour passed, then two. It got very dark but the full Moon was lighting the way. He walked between tall trees; unruly branches were whipping him in the face. He walked through tall grass; fallen wood snagged his feet. He walked through ditches and jumped over springs. He walked and walked and finally, he reached the glade. He pulled a talisman out of his pocket and placed it in the center of the glade; he sat down on the grass and closed his eyes. What should I wish for? thought the Rom. And at this moment an image of a horse appeared in his mind. A bay horse with a long mane and kind eyes. It was neighing and stomping its feet. The Rom clearly heard neighing. Was it true or did it only seem true to him? He opened his eyes and thanked Veshitko Dad. Then he turned his head and looked. Behind him there stood a fine horse, exactly as he had imagined it. The Rom jumped on the horse and, elated, galloped back to the taboro.

While I was studying at a university in Russia, I lived in a dorm. It was a sixteen-floor building with two elevators that never worked. I lived on the fourteenth floor. The dorm didn't have heating or hot water. Often, there wasn't even cold water. During the winter, I would walk downstairs, fill a bucket with snow, and walk upstairs, fourteen floors up.

I shared a tiny room (two beds and a table) with a student from Greece. Long ago, the dorm had a working garbage chute. Every floor had an opening in the wall for garbage. The chute dropped all the way to the first floor and into a large garbage bin. But either the garbage bin was never emptied or the chute got clogged up on one of the floors, because the garbage chute stopped working and no one fixed the problem. There was no other garbage bin next to the dorm, so the students began piling the garbage next to the chute opening, right on the floor, in hopes that someday, someone would clean it up. This day never came. The abundance of garbage attracted cockroaches. There were so many of them on top of each other that I couldn't see one of the walls in our tiny kitchen/corridor. During the night, they crawled on the ceiling and sometimes fell down on us in bed. The beds already had fleas, and I guess the cockroaches wanted some company. During the day, cockroaches could fall in a plate of soup or on our heads. They loved the kitchen. The kitchen/corridor was only six feet by four feet, and when the electric stove was on, it warmed up the space around it and the cockroaches loved the warmth and gathered there. All the other rooms were very cold. During the winter, leftover water in a glass would turn into ice.

The classrooms at the university also didn't have heating. During the lectures, my pen would freeze and I had to warm it up by writing on my palm. My palms would turn black from ink. People don't need to stay warm all of the time. The Romani know that cold is very healing in moderation. When I reached my personal limit for enduring the cold, I would head for one of the major city libraries because it had heating. I spent hours there. Cold made me a straight A student.

I was studying in St. Petersburg when the Soviet Union fell apart. Suddenly, even the bad food disappeared from the stores. We received food stamps that could be exchanged for a pack of noodles. We would stand in line for hours, out in the cold, grasping the food stamps in our hands, so that they wouldn't get stolen from our purses or pockets. Soon I hated noodles. Several years later when I came to America and my college advisor took me to an Italian restaurant, I couldn't hide my disappointment: anything but noodles!

But I didn't know then that I would find myself in America. I didn't know yet that it could become real, but I dreamed about it. No matter how hard my life had been, I was happy because I did a lot of traveling. Mind traveling. When I read about a place, I put myself there. When I stood in line to wait for food, I transported myself elsewhere.

Look around. What do you see? The walls of your house? The couch you are sitting on? What do you hear? The street noise outside? The rustle of leaves? What do you feel? The sadness from a recent argument? Now think about a beach instead. Walk barefoot on the warm sand, look up into the blue sky, listen to the sound of the waves, feel complete happiness. Imagine in detail the sensation of sand in your toes. Smell the sea.

You have just traveled to the beach. Traveled in your mind. If you felt happy there, on the beach in your mind, this feeling will move into your real life. Some day you *will* travel to the beach that you imagined in real life. The expectation of this wonderful moment will enrich your life and make it colorful. And you can mind travel anytime and anywhere as much as you like. No passport or visa required.

Mind traveling is a great tool to change your focus from negative to positive. I remember one day I was walking on the gray carpet of a hospital floor. The long corridor seemed to never end. It was so depressing that I knew I had to do something right away to change my mood or I'd slip from my happy state.

I begin imagining that there was green lush grass under my feet. I picture this green grass with detail. I begin imagining exactly how tall the grass was, I begin "looking" for different hues of green. I try to remember what the smell of the cut grass is like and place it in the corridor with me. I imagine that the ceiling turns into the sky and the walls become mountains. With each step, the smile on my face grows wider. There is a stranger coming toward me. I smile in greeting. He smiles back at me, puzzled. Maybe he is trying to figure out if he had met me somewhere and just didn't remember who I was. I let it be a mystery. I keep walking and my posture becomes straighter. I begin singing a song in my head. Mind. Magic. The brain does not know the difference between the real world and imagination. This power allows us to create our own reality.

One time when I was reading my journal, I found a description of mind traveling I had done in St. Petersburg. During a particularly difficult time, I couldn't travel in my mind directly to a happy place. I had to start in a place of sadness and then move elsewhere from there.

I read in my journal, "I saw an endless field. I saw myself walking alone in this field. A very cold wind was blowing hard and I didn't have warm clothes. I didn't know how far I needed to go before I would find shelter. I was freezing and thinking there would be no help. Yet I kept walking and hoping for a miracle. Finally, I came to the seashore. There was a boat waiting for me. I stepped inside the boat and it took me to a beautiful island. It was such a paradise there: the weather was warm, the people were friendly, and I began feeling so wonderful, so relaxed. Time slowed down, just like the turtles that were abundant on the beach. This feeling of slowness and warmth began in my mind and spread to my body. No matter what happens to us, I thought, help is always around the corner, we just need to 'keep walking' and not give up. And that by imagining a place that is a paradise for us, we will actually create it in our lives." Many years later I found out that American Indians call North America the Turtle Island. What I imagined as a way to cope with difficult times became true as I lived in a place that provided me with that kind of peace.

The Magic Keys

There are many ways to go about mind traveling. You can imagine a long corridor with lots of doors to your left and right. All doors are closed at first, but you have a sturdy ring of keys in your hand. You open the first door to your left. You walk into a greenhouse full of beautiful blooming flowers. You look at roses, orchids, and daisies. Where is your favorite flower? Find it. Spend as much time as you like smelling flowers and looking at butterflies and enjoying the feeling of the lush greenery. Then go back to the corridor.

Open the second door, the one to your right. You'll see several tables full of berries and exotic fruit. Taste them all. Look, there are the fruit trees. Climb them and pick all kinds of fruit. Now go back to the corridor. Open the third door – to your right or to your left, it doesn't matter. The third room displays precious stones. Notice the different sizes, shapes, and colors of the stones. Hold bright cut crystals high against the sunlight streaming through a window to see the rainbow reflections dance in the room behind you. Look at amethyst, ruby, blue topaz, and other stones. They are big and heavy. Each one has a story to tell. Each gives you a unique energy. I "created" these rooms for you because I like green houses, fruit, and natural stones and crystals. You can create your own rooms full of things that you like and visit them any time you wish. Remember that your thoughts are the magic keys that can open any door in the Universe.

Practice mind traveling by going to your "magic place." If you don't have this place in mind yet, create it and travel there during difficult times. A client of mine taught this skill to her mother who was dying of breast cancer. As her mother sat in an exquisite garden on one of her last trips, she spent hours memorizing the size and design of the steep garden built into a hillside. She studied the trees, shrubs, and blooming flowers. She read the inscriptions and enjoyed the statuary. On her deathbed she would close her eyes and smile, returning to the garden she had created in her mind. It gave her peace and joy.

Before I go to bed, I always do the following: I relax and take a few deep breaths as if I am smelling a big, beautiful flower. Then I think of something that I love with all my heart. It may be a person, an animal, or a place in nature. I then feel the emotion of love, getting stronger and stronger, filling my body like a bright light, then filling the whole room, and eventually filling the whole house. When I feel the energy hold itself, I relax and drift into sleep in a wonderful energy field that surrounds me until I wake.

When I was a girl, I was afraid of being alone in the dark. My mind would draw up the scariest of pictures which then felt so real. After I learned to surround myself with this beautiful light, I stopped being afraid of the darkness. Even better, I now have wonderful dreams while I sleep. And if my window is open and the wind gently blows into the room, moving the curtains, I imagine that these are my Angels coming to visit me, creating the wind with their wings. The feeling it creates in the room is truly sacred!

Mind traveling can be not only pleasant, but also very powerful. It can be the last resort when everything else fails.

I'll never forget one of my trips from Estonia to America. I got sick on the day I had to leave. As I was entering the plane, I began feeling a headache. I took a pill, but as we were getting higher and higher into the sky, the headache kept getting stronger and stronger. I took stronger pills, but they simply did not help. The pain became excruciating. I took the maximum number of pills I could take, but I had to spend many more hours on the plane. I began looking out the window, thinking that the blood vessels in my head were going to rupture. I wanted to "jump out" of my body. I was looking at the white clouds, desperately searching for solution. I was in a panic. Just when I thought I could not suffer any longer, I closed my eyes and imagined myself next to a small pond in the mountains. *This pond has healing water*, I thought. I imagined jumping into this pond and going deep under the water. I pretended that I could breathe under the water. I kept telling myself that this water was magical, that it could take away my pain and even give me vitality. I emerged from under the water and sat on the edge of the pond. I called it "The Pool of Youth." I saw myself in beautiful white clothes, sitting next to the pond, smiling peacefully. There was no more pain and when I caught a glimpse of myself in the lavatory mirror, I definitely looked younger! My headache had stopped and I realized the true power of imagination to heal and delight.

You can practice mind traveling while sitting still with your eyes closed, or you can practice it while moving your body with your eyes open like in the Romani energy exercises I'll share with you. I've used them in conjunction with other healing work. I once went to a workshop where we were guided through some deep, negative emotions. It drained our spirit so much! But at the end of the workshop, we pretended to splash each other with water, just like kids splash each other in the pool. The scene was hilarious! A bunch of grown-ups "splashing" each other with invisible water. We left the workshop feeling energized and definitely younger. I amplified this work with what I know from Roma ways and it changed my world.

If you are sad, notice your body language, posture, and facial expression. Now change it. Which body language brings you a feeling of peace? A feeling of power? Imagine that you are a king or a queen and then try to behave like one. You will notice that your thoughts and your mood will change right away. Reclaim your adult imagination as a part of your freedom. Live with the power to create your life as you choose it.

Problem: You are not living your dream; you are not following your passion.

Solution: Think about your dream or your passion every day. Create it in your mind with as many details as possible. Think about it first thing in the morning and last thing at night. Take small steps to make your dream or passion a reality. You must first create it in your mind and then in your life.

A Word is Not a Bird: Once It Flies Away, You Can't Catch It

It happened a long time ago, during the olden times. One taboro was traveling through an unknown land. It was time to make a camp and Roma set up their tents close to a small town. One of Roma says, "I'll walk to the town to explore this and that." And he set off on foot early in the morning. As he approached the town, he saw a tall wall, as tall as a mountain. Right next to the wall, he saw a crowd of people. The Rom walked closer to the crowd and heard a heated discussion, only he could not understand a word. In the middle of the crowd, there was a richly dressed man showing several gold coins from his palm. The crowd got louder, but the Rom didn't understand that the people were saying this: "Hey, rich man, put away your gold coins, don't you see how tall the wall is? No one in the world would be able to climb it, and the one who tries will be badly hurt." However, a few volunteers began climbing the wall. What were they talking about? thought the Rom.

Maybe the gold coins are the reward to the person who climbs the wall first? And he also began climbing the wall without looking down. After some time, he was on top of the wall, but he was the only one who had made it. Others, having heard about how dangerous the wall was, either turned back half-way or fell. Only the Rom, who did not understand what people were saying, made it to the very top. He got the gold coins and happily returned to his taboro. You see? What you believe becomes so.

THE POWERFUL MAGIC OF WORDS

I have created many exercises to feel the positive power of words. One of them is to pick any positive word - for example, *excitement*. Now find as many related words as you can: elation, delight, pleasure, enchantment, ecstasy, bliss, thrill, and even seventh heaven! Start using a variety of positive words any chance you get. *I am delighted to see you! I am thrilled! I am in seventh heaven!* Use your more varied, powerful, and interesting words at home, at work, and most importantly, say them in your own head. Charming!

Once, I wrote several "happy" words on pieces of paper and placed them in different parts of my house. Marvelous, miraculous, spectacular, splendid, fabulous, breathtaking, remarkable, luminous. Later, I would accidentally find them and smile.

The Romani language is very colorful and expressive. It is full of idioms, metaphors, and blessings. You will often hear "Let God give you good luck" or phrases such as, "A warm-hearted word is better than an expensive present" and "Let your health last one hundred years" or "My blood is boiling!" and "Wit without tongue is like the face without the eyes." This is a powerful use of language as everyday speach, and it enlivens conversations.

There are also ways to deepen communication through chanting. From the time people spoke their first word and for thousands and thousands of years afterwards, everyone has known the power of a chant. A chant is a combination of words that create positive energy. I have a list of chants that I use when my mind drifts off into negative thinking:

> I am the healthiest person on Earth!
> The Universe sends me a generous gift!
> I enjoy every second of life!
> I deserve very best in this wonderful world!

As a reminder to use my chants, every time I am drinking water, I say to myself, "This water brings me health, happiness, and love." When I go outside, I look at the blue skies and say, "I am breathing in joy, energy, and beauty, and I am breathing out fatigue, irritation, and pain."

I even rhyme some chants:

> Every day I'm getting younger,
> Every day I'm getting stronger.

I play with…

> I love the world and the world loves me,
> I love the Earth and the Earth loves me,

I love the people and the people love me,
I love the animals and the animals love me,
I love the trees and the trees love me.

Then I add anything that comes to my mind:

Gifts of healing, magic power flow right to me.

Then I repeat or sing these lines many, many times. I sing my chants when I am jogging, when I am driving, when I am doing dishes. I know it is up to me to add magic to my days and nights.

Chants work better when you say them out loud. In the beginning, you will feel silly saying things like "I am the healthiest person on Earth," especially if you are currently sick. But just give it a try. The results will amaze you. Find a place where no one can hear you and just say it. You will notice that saying positive chants will make you smile. Chant while looking in the mirror. Look yourself in the eyes and say "I am beautiful!" My favorite chants are:

I love my life!
I love the Universe!
This is such a beautiful place!

If you can't find a place where no one will hear you, whisper your chants or write them down on a piece of paper. Chanting in your head is not as powerful because if you think, "I am happy," your mind may say, "No, you're not." The mind is impressed by action. I dare you to go into the forest and scream as loud as you can, "I love my life!!!" Then compare it to saying it in your head. You will notice the difference in your body and soul.

In the very beginning, you don't have to believe in what you are saying. Just repeat the chants. You will become an expert once you say a chant *knowing* that as you say it, so it is.

Here are some old Romani chants:

Bad weather slips away, gives the Sun its way.
Happiness walks inside; trouble walks outside.

Problem: You feel unhappy.
Solution: Track the words you are thinking and speaking. Notice how many words are optimistic and positive and how many words are pessimistic and negative. Pinch yourself each time you use a depressing word. Change it into an encouraging one. The words you are thinking and speaking create your life.

One king was looking for a bride for his son. He had only one condition: the girl should be loving and caring, with a kind heart and a pure soul. He met many girls on his path and selected two for consideration. Both seemed perfect. How to make the final decision without making a mistake? How to find out if one was pretending to be kind but was evil inside?

The king turned to an old Shuvihani, a Gypsy healer, for advice. Shuvihani said, "Invite both girls to a formal dinner and ask them to tell something about themselves. Then just watch and observe what happens in the room."

The king followed the advice. He invited many guests to his castle; both girls were among the guests. This and that happened, and soon it was time to find out what was so. He asked the first girl to tell something about herself. She began to speak, and after each word an ugly toad jumped from her mouth. The servants were barely able to catch them all. The king turned to the second girl and asked her to tell something about herself. She began to speak, and after each word a beautiful flower dropped from her mouth. Soon, the entire ballroom was filled with a delicate fragrance. Now, who would you pick as the bride?

Whether you are aware of this or not, what falls out of your mouth has a particular energy. On some level you know this, and others do too. Notice that when someone tells the truth from their heart, people lean in to hear more, and when someone is lying—even if they seem convincing on the surface—people in the room can sense the lack of integrity. Energy is what matters, and we know when it is bad and when it is good.

Turn Every Bad Day into a Good Day to Live a Good Life

A Gypsy woman was returning from her trip to the city back to her taboro. She hoped to get some food for her family in exchange for fortune-telling. Unfortunately, it started to snow hard and she didn't find any customers. On her way back, the snow was covering her eyes and she lost her way. She saw a warm fire in the distance and walked toward it. Around the fire there sat twelve men, young and old. The Gypsy greeted the men and asked if she could warm up next to their fire. The youngest man cleared the space and said, "Sure, have a seat, it's January, the worst month of all, don't you think?" The woman sat down and said, "Thank you, you are so kind. But I would disagree with you. January is not bad at all. It's the beginning of the New Year, new hopes, new dreams. It is time for Christmas (*in Russia, Christmas is celebrated in the beginning of January). It is time for bringing families together, time for joy and celebration." Then an older man said, "February must be the worst month of all then." "I am sorry to disagree with you too," responded the woman. "New life is stirring inside the Earth during February. Without February, there would be no March. And let me tell you about March " The woman went on to describe each month of the year and had praise and love for all of them. Then the oldest man grinned and said he had a gift for the Gypsy. He gave her a small sack and asked her not to open it until she got home. The woman thanked the men, took the sack, and headed home. The snow stopped and she easily found her taboro. She then opened the sack and found twelve gold coins in it, one from each month of the year.

I stepped into an elevator in Los Angeles, a city where the sun shines brightly most days of the warm year. A woman with a sour expression remarked to the strangers in the elevator, "Oh it's so cold." The day was slightly overcast and there was a slight breeze. If this woman complained about the weather in one of the most temperate places on earth, imagine the level of complaint she was bringing to everything and everyone else in her life. What must it be like to work with her, be her friend, be married to her? I sent her love and a smile. "Aren't we lucky," I said, "to enjoy such weather!"

When clients are stuck in complaint, I invite them to instead be creative. We identify the areas in life they are complaining about and find the ways they can bring Gypsy wisdom to making magic out of them. Often the largest treasure is buried underneath the scariest dragon. Many times the map of complaint becomes the path to joy. It is often the smallest things that show the way.

One day, I was walking to a café for lunch. It was a warm spring day. There were dark clouds in the sky, so I grabbed my jacket "just in case it rained." A few minutes passed and I noticed that the sky was getting darker and darker. Suddenly, there came a strong wind and it started to rain and then hail, hard. I put on my jacket, wishing I had an umbrella and hunched against the weather, fighting it and holding complaint in my heart. I kept walking. All I could think of was that it was cold. Then I saw a man holding a little girl in his arms. She did not have a jacket. She was wearing a t-shirt and he held her close to give her more warmth. She wriggled in his arms, clapped her hands, and merrily shouted, "Daddy, Daddy, let's make snowballs!" In response to her delight, I smiled, forgot about the cold, and learned my lesson. The weather didn't change. I changed my perspective. No matter what happens in my life, I will chose my perspective and I will choose to love my life.

What are you bringing a dark attitude to that can instead be turned into, "Let's make snowballs!" If you find yourself becoming cranky in rush hour traffic, make sure you have music you love to provide a private concert in your car. Don't enjoy cleaning up the kitchen after dinner? Make it a fun ritual by adding something you love to the task— listening to something wonderful that is inspiring, or to a comedian who makes you laugh. We only become stuck in "bad" days or in tasks we imagine unpleasant if we stop bringing liveliness and creativity to every small and large thing we do. Be creative and joy will flow!

These large and small daily decisions are what create the quality of your life. Learn from what you observe and what the world and her people show you. Watch for the magic found in the lessons unfolding around you.

Every person has their own level of perception, the way they look at the world. One person will go outside, glance at a weed, and their mood will be spoiled for the rest of the day. Another person will look at the same weed, bend to look closer at the tiny leaves, and will see the drops of dew and how the rays of the Sun are reflected in it. The mood of this grateful person will be such that they will want to sing and dance for the rest of the day. Which of these people will be blessed by the Kingdom?

Do you understand that you are creating your reality? Have you heard about the "law" that says, "If something can go wrong, it will"?

I have recently realized that it is not the law, it is a test of your energy level and how much you are willing to create your life. If trouble seems to follow you around, your energy is low and it attracts negative events into your life. An act of kindness and selflessness immediately raises your energy, and as a result bad things will stop happening to you so frequently.

You also have the power to change your attitude toward little mishaps—think of them as a small test only—and they will stop happening. There will be much less "bad luck" in your life if you put yourself in charge of generating your own good luck. It's impossible to have all good luck all the time though. Remember, we have to accept life as it is in order to have peace. All of us will experience bad luck in some moments. Both good and bad luck are present in life at all times. Life is not a paradise, the Kingdom does contain "bad things." Even when your luck is good, you will see people around you who are suffering.

There are always illnesses, accidents, floods, fires, earthquakes, and tragedies. When we see people suffer, we can choose to feel compassion and to do everything we can to support and help them while at the same time recognize that nothing is wrong with the world. Life is made up of all of these things.

When little misfortunes do happen, accept them with gratitude. In Russia, it is considered good luck to find a hair in your soup or to break a cup. A little "bad" thing is believed to keep the larger ones away in the way that a small earthquake can release tension in the earth so that a big one may become less likely.

Be thankful when you have a flat tire – you didn't get into a car accident. Be thankful if you get in a minor car accident – you didn't get hurt. I even know of a woman who, in the midst of a serious car accident as many of her bones were being shattered, was thinking, "I am grateful this is not going to kill me and I will use the healing of my physical injuries to heal my life." She was grateful for a potentially deadly car accident in the moment she experienced it! You will not be surprised to hear that she is now an amazing healer.

If you focus on little or big misfortunes, they will ruin your life and you will be a victim in life's dramas. If you accept misfortune and don't get angry or complain, the biggest misfortunes will walk past you. And if you suffer big misfortunes, you can embrace those as well as an extreme part of life and surrender to what is happening. Many times people look back at a time years before as one of the BEST times of their lives when, at the time, they were actually experiencing it as the worst. Give yourself time to understand your experiences. Let life unfold itself, and give yourself the gift of unraveling the mysteries of life slowly.

Choose Your Joy

We were not created to be in a constant state of happiness. But if you are not happy most of the time, don't blame the events or people in your life; choose to change your perspective.

Our thoughts and feelings determine our lives. Not our words – we can easily say what we don't think is true. Not our actions – we often do what others expect of us. It is what we think and feel that matters. Every second. Every minute. Every thought and feeling counts. A thought, released by your mind, immediately becomes a part of your energy field. A feeling, released by your heart, immediately becomes a part of your soul. Negative thoughts and feelings attract negative events into your life while positive thoughts and feelings attract positive events. When we think about the same thing over and over again, we give the thoughts our energy. When we feel a certain way over and over again, we create our destiny. Our thoughts and feelings are like horses that gallop to the land where wishes come true.

When you create powerful wishes and bring courage to difficult times, your ability to be joyful increases. You have the capacity to surround yourself with a community of like-minded people. Use that power. When people band together in times of stress, difficult times can actually be fun. I know of a neighborhood that organizes shared meals and where people stay in touch because of a terrible flood that caused them a great deal of loss and pain years ago. They had to all band together to endure something very traumatic, and guess what happened? They loved and served each other and went from living side by side without any connection for decades to being a real community. This sense of connection can be created without needing the pressure of a difficult situation to generate it, so long as you are willing to engage the people around you in bold and loving action. What can you do to help your neighborhood connect? How can you *be* a neighbor so that there is life and love where you live?

When you walk in the world with love, magic follows you as if petals are falling from flowers above to cover the path before you. Compassion for people in the world is like a special talisman of love and protection. We put amulets and charms in our pockets when we go out into the world. We look at the world with beautiful eyes. We say positive magical words. We eat healthy food. We do everything we can to create a beautiful life and then, when we have done as much as we can, we surrender to what life does to us and love life no matter what happens. In Romani culture, if something bad happens to us or our family or in the world around us, we have great strength to face it. We stand up straight and tall and walk right into the trouble. This is possible because we have lived so much of our time in peace and joy. As you create magic in everyday life, you will dial up the good luck surrounding you so that it is with you much more of the time. This is possible. I've done it, and I've taught others to do it too.

Remember that to maintain a happy state, you can't let yourself be upset by little mishaps, by small annoyances like being stuck in traffic, or else more serious problems will be attracted to you. Laugh at little mishaps and inconveniences and small hurts and transgressions. Think of someone to forgive, give a random act of kindness, and watch the good luck period in your life begin anew. Create a rule for your life that says, "If something good can happen, I'm certain it will!"

Filling Your Energy Reserves

Each time you think a negative thought or feel a negative emotion, your body gets tense. This tension can be physical, mental, emotional, or even spiritual. Over time, this will deplete your energy reserves. On the contrary, each time you think a positive thought or feel a positive emotion, your body gets relaxed, and this increases your energy reserves.

The best way to relieve physical tension and replace fresh, new energy in your body and spirit is through movement. The best way to relieve mental tension is by mind traveling to your "magical place." The best way to relieve emotional tension is to do something that brings you joy. The best way to relieve spiritual tension is gratitude.

Once I was planning a vacation to Hawaii. I read a few stories about local healers. I was particularly attracted to those specializing in lomilomi – a highly spiritual, transformational form of massage. A local Hawaiian healer would start the session with a prayer, connecting to the One, and then chant during the massage or talk about healing herbs and remedies for a specific condition. These traditional healers spend a lifetime learning the laws of vibration, spoken word, healing touch, and nature. They pray as they harvest the plants they use in their ceremony. One famous practitioner described it as "gathering the vibration of the plentiful." Someone was offering lomilomi at a local hotel. I couldn't wait to try it.

When I arrived in Hawaii, I was about to call the hotel to make an appointment, but I had an uneasy feeling. All of a sudden, I wasn't excited about it anymore. I had to make an effort to pick up the phone. My intuition is very strong, and this uneasiness was a sign for me not to make the appointment. *What could be wrong with lomilomi?* I thought. I didn't listen to my intuition, was stubborn, and picked up the phone anyway. I called the Spa at the hotel and booked an appointment.

Several hours later, I walked into the Spa and was greeted ... by a Caucasian man who was too young to have studied the decades required by traditional practitioners. I tried to relax on the massage table, hoping that the Hawaiian traditional massage could be taught to non-locals. No, it was a regular massage, and a rather bad and expensive one. I was literally soaking in oil, and the energy of the experience was completely off. I was irritated rather than relaxed. It was so disappointing! The massage was not even close to what I had intended to experience. I also lost valuable time that I could have spent on other activities. I had to stop repeating over and over again, "I wish I hadn't made this appointment." I knew right away that I had to get rid of this disappointment quickly so that it wouldn't spoil the rest of the day or even the rest of the week! I had learned a valuable lesson—to listen more closely to the push and pull of my intuitive messages.

The best way to reset my energy was to swim in the ocean. I knew that water, especially salt water, not only cleanses our physical bodies but also removes negative emotions from our spirit. I ran into the ocean with as much passion and power as if tigers were chasing after me. As I swam I thought about someone who could not afford to ever come to Hawaii, someone who would never have any type of massage done, ever. I instantly felt a sense of gratitude, and the negativity of that experience was washed away with the waves.

Disappointment is a very strong negative emotion. If it hangs around you, the energy attracts even more disappointment. In addition to washing it away, I decided to replace disappointment with a strong positive emotion. After I reset my energy in the water to deep gratitude, I went into the best restaurant on the island. My eyes ate the breathtaking sunset, I enjoyed delicious food and appreciated how lucky I was to be there. As soon as I felt great again, the most unusual thing happened. I ordered a dessert with an unfamiliar name without knowing what it was. The chef rolled a cart to my table. He put a plate in front of me and with a fruit and a knife created a beautiful flower on the plate right in front of my eyes. He was making this edible art with such passion and attention to detail that I enjoyed it profoundly. It was a masterpiece! I had been blessed and my energy and magic were high again.

The tension was gone and I felt completely relaxed. The world suddenly became friendly and bright. Most of us forget what it's like to be completely relaxed. Physically, you feel as if your body is light and flexible. Your movements are slow and calm, your gaze is kind and soft. Mentally, you either don't have any thoughts (without any effort on your part) or your thoughts are very clear. Emotionally, you feel on top of the world! You feel inspiration and the power to accomplish anything you wish. You smile or even giggle for no reason. Spiritually, you feel connected to all, everything and everyone. During this time of total relaxation, healing takes place simultaneously on all levels of the body/mind/spirit.

In the same way I did, you too have the personal power to choose to be happy here and now—any second you choose, no matter what happened in the past. Gypsies live in the present moment. The future is not here yet, so why worry about it. There is also no use in regretting the past. It's done and over with. Now is all we have, and it is precious.

Many people postpone life. They think, "I will live fully when..." When the kids are older, when I get a new job, after I lose weight, or whatever nonsense they invent to delay joy. Yet time passes and one condition they set up is replaced by for another. Life passes by like a train while they wait on the track, and they feel they are living a not-right-life, waiting for the perfect moment to embrace a new life but never finding that perfect moment. Now is all you have. The past is gone and the future is the sum of your "nows." You can create it as you wish.

Pulling In Happiness from Nature

There is a way to work with your brain to get it to do what you want in a different manner than you might expect. You can tell yourself a "lie" briefly: a lie that quickly becomes a truth. If right now you don't feel happy, PRETEND to be happy. Borrow the wisdom from the world around you. It helps a lot if you imagine that you are some part of nature. Play this game with your friends when you are confronted by unhappiness: pretend to be a flower, the Sun, a big wave. How would you behave? What kind of thoughts or emotions would you have? Facial expressions? Body language? How would you relate to those around you? Try it; it will bring you a lot of fun. Or just imagine what you would feel if you were a tree. I connect so deeply with trees that I love them like family.

I am always amazed and delighted by the trees in the spring. There they are, leafless. One day passes, another, and another. Nothing looks different. Then, all of a sudden, there is a subtle light-green cloud surrounding the tree. It is growing quietly and quickly. That's how you will change. That's how your life will change when you learn to live in the now. Life will open up her beautiful secrets.

Romanies have one of the most hurtful pasts as a people. But we also have mastered the skill of forgetting it. No matter what has caused you great sorrow in the past, leave it there and focus on creating a beautiful future for yourself in the now. Grow!

When you are doing something, anything, think about what you are doing in a positive way. When you are eating, think about the food on your plate with gratitude. Smell it, taste all the different flavors, look at the rainbow of colors on your plate, and enjoy every bite. Don't think about plans for tomorrow and don't replay the events of the past. Just think about the food on your plate. This will bring you emotional and physical benefits as you eat. You will feel great, and the food will feel your appreciation and will digest much better because part of what you are eating is your own personal joy.

A Last Day

Celebrate every breath. Live as if this is your last day on earth. When someone asked me to describe what my last day would be like, here is what I said. "On the last day of my life, I will be in nature. I will breathe in the fresh air as if I am drinking it through my nose. I will hug the trees, roll down the hills, then I will rest on the ground, looking up at the sky. I will walk through the streets. I will smile and say, "Hello dear friends," to strangers passing. I will say, 'Isn't it a lovely day?'" But why wait until the last day? I am going to do that right now!

Don't drink life with small sips; gulp it all up and swallow it. Don't pretend to be someone else. Open up to any and all experiences and live as fully as you can, every moment of life. Here is your secret to happiness. We are all Masters; we all can create miracles.

Here's a magical way to create. Imagine a door to a beautiful room and take the key to the lock in your hand. Your Guardian Angel is waiting for you in that room. All you need to do is find the right key to open the door. Then you can ask your Guardian Angel any wish and your wish will be granted. You just have to open the door. You may say, "I want to see my Guardian Angel, so that I can believe in it." But if the Guardian Angel appeared before you in a physical form like a human being it would not be able to do what it is meant to do – assist you in your wishes in the spiritual realm. Let it be in the magic of the other side of the door helping you in the realm of the unseen. The more positive your thoughts and emotions, the closer you are to your Angel and the faster your wishes will come true. Hurry, hurry to make good deeds out of your everyday actions. They will raise your energy and speed up the realization of your deepest desires.

Another way to raise your energy is to visit sacred places, create sacred things, wear holy objects, and meet holy people. Learn to surround your body with the feeling of sacred and then recreate it at home as well. You are precious and so is your life. Treat it as sacred and magic will unfold.

I really like the word *awe*. Only very small children and very spiritual people tend to look at the world with awe. Feel the difference in tightening your eyes against the world and seeing ugliness and ordinariness. Now look at the world and everything in it with awe, reverence, delight, admiration, and *inspiration*, a word that is translated as the "breath of God." This is the biggest secret of happiness. We all can recreate this feeling. Can you treat every object as sacred? Can you treat every person as holy? I have visited many sacred places to learn and grow, and I have realized that I am able to create a sacred place in my home. It is all about energy. I have learned to master very high energies which I can show you. There are ways to bring nature and natural energies into your house with sacred pieces of wood, stone, and other natural elements and pieces of art that feel sacred. Once, I saw an extraordinary painting by a Russian artist I admire. It was as if the Sun itself had painted the image with its rays. Soft, quiet hues. Sun, dissolved in water. It was an artful representation of the soul and the rays of the heart. This is what sacred feels like to me! As soon as I could, I placed his work in the sacred temple of my home.

You can also watch for the images, objects, and talismans that resonate as powerful for you. Your symbols of a great life can surround you. The magic of creation can be right there—in the palm of your hand.

An Open and Positive Mind

Learn to always keep an open and positive mind. You never know when a miracle is around the corner. You don't want to miss that, so watch for it every day!

Here is a quick test to find out if you have an open and positive mind. Imagine you are walking along a street and see a person flying in the air without anything to support their flight. Do you:

1. Say, "This is not true, because this cannot be true."
2. Think, "I am losing my mind."
3. Observe, "A new magician in town, how fun!"
4. Speculate, "This is probably a Yogi who spent 50 years in a cave mastering this, there is no way I could do it."

5. Celebrate, "Finally, somebody learned how to fly, which means I can do it too!"

If you chose options 1-3, you don't see miracles in your life, you simply screen them out and overlook them. Option 4 – you were conditioned not to believe in yourself. Option 5 – your life is magical every day and you show up ready to be inspired!

Another breakthrough you can have to open up your perceptions of life is this simple realization. Connect with the truth that nobody takes anything with them as they leave this world. We say this, but only when we really understand it does life get brighter. Here's a way to understand this idea down to your bones.

In a time of great sorrow or misfortune, go to a cemetery and read the headstones. An old man who was coughing and smoking a cigarette limped through a graveyard and said, "There are people here who would die to have my cough." Connect with the reality of your own mortality with a smile. Look at your circumstances and say, "At least I'm not dead." Death is an important aspect of Gypsy culture. There are many traditions around death. How we handle possessions and grief are the ones people are most curious about because so many people accumulate things up to the day they die. Romani keep nothing of the person's after they are gone.

When the person dies, there is a very intense grieving process. People scream and sob and don't eat for three days. We turn ourselves over to our grief, and we express our sorrow as we wail and cry out loud and get it completely out of our system. It may seem strange, but the expression of grief is absolutely essential to clearing the energy of what happens next, and it also brings good health because the grief does not get stuck in our bodies to cause disease or illness later on. When someone is buried, the grave is made beautiful, kept clean and well-marked. We bring little gifts to the grave as we would to make a home beautiful and full of magic. People put things in the casket for the person they loved to take on their journey. The family visits the grave often and makes sure it is in good condition. This constant going to the cemetery to take care of these little sacred chores reminds us that life is a gift. It reminds us that material things don't count, only good memories do. And memories are made in the passion of the everyday moment.

While some people are dead on their feet living an ordinary and boring life, others are engaged in it with power and energy. We have a saying, "Don't die before death takes you."

The Shuvihani Journey

I once met a woman of great spiritual power. She called herself a shaman and I could immediately feel her power. I liked her instantly. She had a very soft glow of love surrounding her. She did bodywork, in which energy work is combined with a hot stone massage and aromatherapy. I set up an appointment with her not knowing what to expect. During the massage, I closed my eyes and relaxed. A few minutes later, I saw with my mind's eye a yellow feather. I told my shaman healer about it. She interpreted it this way: "It is a message for you. It has to do with your childhood. You have to find out what it means yourself." I started thinking about my childhood. I couldn't figure out what the message was. I remembered my home town, but did I remember a yellow feather? My town was about eight hundred years old, with castles and towers, brick pavement and horse carts. It had such a magical feeling about it. Wait a minute – I hadn't been there for ages! I missed it. I will go visit my hometown now! As soon as I had that thought, I got a feeling of such joy that I knew it was time to go home. I bought the ticket right away. I arrived anticipating discovering the next piece of the puzzle. Why did I have to come here right now? Who would I meet? What would I learn? I looked attentively at every stranger sitting next to me on the bus. I took time to get to know people and ask them questions. I didn't know yet that the message would come from my childhood friend.

We have been friends since high school and her name is Olga. When I moved to the United States, we would send each other audio tapes with things we wanted to share. Talking on the phone was too expensive and e-mail didn't exist then. When we met up, Olga gave me a book. I thanked her and put the book in my backpack. I was so busy searching for the message about the yellow feather, I didn't have time to read it while I was there. Although I had a great time on my trip, it seemed as if nothing extraordinary had happened. I returned home, satisfied with my travels but unsure if I had connected with the deeper purpose of the trip. I unpacked my bags and for the first time studied the book Olga had given me. It was about making wishes come true by using the power of thoughts! It was just what I needed at the time, and reading it was as if I was receiving a message from the heavens. I read the whole book in a few days. Each page was connected to some part of my soul. I had forgotten how magical my life used to be. This book reminded me that my thoughts have enormous power. I kept the thought of the yellow feather as a guide in my discovery.

I understood that feathers are believed by many magical and indigenous peoples to carry messages to and from higher realms. They can signal new beginnings, flight, or freedom. And I knew that for me yellow was a color linked to a "gut feeling," strong intuition, psychic ability, and also focus.

So in flying around the world to connect with just the right lesson that I needed, I received gifts on more levels than I could count. I began paying attention to what I was thinking about when I was driving my car, hiking, cooking, or cleaning. I became an observer of my own thought patterns. I was shocked to realize that after the skating accident and the long healing process that followed, most of my thinking had been negative! I often thought "What if..." – "What if this goes wrong?" "What if that happens?" and so on. Another pattern was "I should have..." – "I should have done this," "I should have done that..." I hadn't noticed that I had stopped my creative thinking. If thoughts were things, my head was full of trash! I changed this by keeping track of my thoughts throughout the day. Was I complaining or feeling gratitude? Was I anticipating negative or positive events? In the beginning, I didn't have many positive, creative thoughts. No wonder I was missing out on the sparkle and excitement that life had to offer.

I also realized that some of my thinking resembled a radio station. Sometimes I was running my own show, but other times I was just picking up other people's random static in the form of thoughts and ideas, ones that were not necessarily beneficial to me. In time, I learned to distinguish my own thoughts from those I picked up from other people. Thoughts that belong to me seem natural, easy and fun. Other people's negative energies always seem "heavy" and unpleasant, and I learned how not to connect with them. All thanks to a yellow feather.

Problem: You lost your job and your house.
Solution: Gypsies know too well what it is like not to have a job and not to have a house. If this were to affect their spirits, their lives would become one endless road of misery. Use the free time

to learn something new, spend time with your family, explore the nature around you, volunteer, find new friends, and most of all, appreciate the freedom you now have, because soon you will have a job and then you'll be remembering those free days fondly.

One time, a Rom was walking along a meadow. He saw a peasant sitting with his hands around his head and a horse nearby. "What a great horse you have," said the Rom.

The peasant lifted his head; his face filled with sadness. "Oh, my life, my life, my bitter, bitter life," said the peasant, sobbing. "This horse is all I have. I had a house, but it burned to the ground. I have nothing, nothing, just this horse. I am so unhappy. So unhappy."

Hearing these words, the Rom walked towards the horse, jumped on it, and vanished into thin air. The peasant began crying out loud, "Oh, my horse, my horse, what am I to do now?" During that time, the Rom trotted not far away and turned back. He approached the peasant, jumped off the horse, and returned it to the peasant.

Seeing his horse, the peasant could not believe his eyes. He began petting the horse, saying, "My horse, my beloved horse. I am the happiest man in the entire world!"

The One Who is Scared of Beng is Not a Rom

The belief in beng, or the devil or a dark force in the world, is one of the key beliefs in Romani culture. Everything evil is associated with beng. Sometimes he actively participates in the life of the taboro, causing bad luck, misfortune, disasters, all kinds of trouble, and ill health. Think of beng as collective negative forces. They are playing a game with you and their goal is to make you miserable. Your goal is to outwit them and not let them drive you into sadness or despair.

Imagine a bad event in your life. Let's say it's a flat tire. You are standing on a highway, all alone, with a flat tire and no help. On top of that, it begins to rain, hard. Your first reaction is to get upset. Wait, imagine for a minute that a little furry devil with a long tail, a couple of horns and a wicked grin crawled under your car and punched a hole in your tire. He is now hiding somewhere close by, waiting for you to show any signs of disturbance. Nothing will make him happier than having you become upset, so instead, with a wide smile on your face and the necessary tools in your hands, you bravely step under the rain and, singing a happy song, calmly change your flat tire. You won. You have the power.

The beng was still thinking. His tail was drooping in disappointment, for he couldn't think of a way to destroy those Gypsies. One time he used his evil power to strike their camp with lightning. Gypsies smiled and used it to light a campfire and then gathered around it singing and dancing. Another day he caused a heavy downpour soaking the Gypsies and all their belongings. They took it as a sign that it was time to travel to a different place, cheering each other as they moved along in the mud to find a better place. The beng studied Gypsies day and night, searching for some weakness. He decided that if he couldn't destroy the whole taboro, he would destroy them one by one.

One day a Romny (Gypsy woman) was making a new pillow. Beng turned himself into a goose and waddled right by her. The woman needed just a handful more feathers, so she plucked the goose and finished her pillow. The first night sleeping on the new pillow, she had terrible nightmares. She woke up in a cold sweat and was not able to fall asleep again. She consulted a Shuvihani who told her to take a big stick and give her pillow a beating. As the woman hit the pillow with all her might, beng felt the striking of the stick on his back. He moaned and screamed, turned and twisted, unable to avoid the strike of the stick. He ran to the Romny and kneeled down before her, begging her to stop hitting the pillow. Gasping, the Romny realized that it was a cursed pillow and so she threw it into the fire. Beng's feathers caught fire. He ran away and jumped into a swamp. Rumor has it, he still has some burnt feathers. You see, you can always cope with whatever comes your way.

Problem: Misfortune keeps happening in your life.
Solution: Don't let beng crash your spirit. Find a new way to celebrate life and focus on the little things that go well. Refuse to give in to the wicked games where the sole purpose is to make you miserable. Take control of the situation and turn it into something positive. Beng will leave you alone and the misfortunes will stop.

Nine

OPENING YOUR HEART

Whole in His Pocket, a Rom Sings a Song

One time, a Romani family asked a wealthy merchant if they could spend the winter in his house. The merchant lived alone in a very big house, but he allowed them to live only in his shed. The merchant enjoyed large amounts of food for breakfast, lunch, and dinner while the Romani family had only a simple dinner once a day. The merchant had lots of money while the Romani family didn't have a single penny. The merchant had only one problem   he didn't sleep well during the night. He turned and tossed around in his bed, falling asleep only by early morning and rising tired every day. When the

Romani family woke up well rested, they sang songs. They would sing so loudly and the songs were so joyful that the merchant sent his servant to bring one of the Romanies to him.

"How is your life?" asks the merchant.

"Everything is well," says the rom.

"Tell me, Gypsy, why do you sing every morning? Is your life that happy?"

"It is very happy indeed. I have a beautiful wife, wonderful children, and a great horse. What else does a man need?"

"Do you have any money?"

"No, I've never had any money and don't have a penny now."

"Well then," says the merchant, "I see you are a good man, here   this is a sack full of money. Take it."

The rom took the sack and ran back to the shed. From that day, the rom stopped sleeping well at night and stopped singing in the morning. Was he afraid that someone would steal the money? Was he thinking what to do with the money? One day passed, then another. Finally, the rom returned the sack to the merchant. "Take it back," he said. "My sleep and my songs are worth more than all the money in the world."

came to America with two small bags and I was happy with what I had. All my possessions fit into these two bags (one of them was my feather pillow, highly valued by Romanies and my close companion for many years by then). During my first few days in the United States, I noticed that Americans wore a new outfit every day. I was confused; I couldn't understand why. Certainly it didn't get dirty after just one day. In Russia, I had two outfits for warm weather and two outfits for cold weather, and I washed each when it had been worn a few times and had become dirty.

I began walking around my new neighborhood, admiring beautiful houses. Once in a while I would stop in front of a house and just stare. An old gentleman walked out of the house I was staring at and asked if he could help me. I said that I had just arrived and was surprised by the beautiful houses I saw in the neighborhood. I asked if I could see what his house looked like on the inside. He didn't mind. When I entered the house, I saw so much furniture, so many carpets, vases, pictures, and so on. There were many things, but I could immediately sense that the house and the contents of the house were stagnant, unhappy. The house could barely breathe. When he opened a door into one of the bedrooms and said, "This is my daughter's room," I was speechless. The room was overflowing: hundreds of stuffed animals, clothes and shoes everywhere, jewelry on every surface, books, videotapes, and lots and lots of things. She would have needed hundreds of bags to pack her things! The room was a complete mess; none of the valuable possessions were being cared for and loved. This would be unacceptable to Gypsies. I thanked the old gentleman and left the house. Now I knew how someone could wear a new outfit every day – there was not enough space in the closet to hold the number of clothes.

Everything Has a Soul

Romanies have a different attitude towards *thing*s. We experience that each thing has a soul. It is very important where each thing came from, whether it was made with love (mass production is frowned upon because it doesn't have soul) and what kind of energy it carries (for example, cotton, silk, linen, and wool clothes have high energy; synthetic clothes drain your energy).

I don't drink from an ordinary cup. Instead, I have a hand-made creation that can be used as a cup but that is also a piece of art. My skirt looks like the ocean suspended in time. My blouse looks like a field of flowers. Everything I own inspires me and fills me with admiration. If you have something that you don't love or don't use, this thing becomes "sick" and negatively affects the energy of your home. Things like it when you take care of them. You have to touch everything you own frequently and with love. Inanimate objects understand the emotion of love very well. Here are my two favorite examples:

A copier at my work suddenly stopped working. It was a new copier and my administrative assistant could not figure out what was wrong. We had to meet a deadline for an important project, and I had to make several copies right away. My administrative assistant asked me what she should do, and I told her to stroke the copier gently with her hand and tell it how much she loved it and appreciated all it did for us. Needless to say, she laughed at my "joke" and asked me again what she should do. As she watched me, I approached the copier with a smile and began stroking it with my hand as if it were my pet. I thanked it for its hard work and asked politely to keep doing a great job. I explained that we needed it to do its job right then and explained why. I then pushed the start button. It worked! Do you think my assistant was amazed? No. With a straight face she told me that it was a coincidence.

When a favorite and rare music CD of mine was ruined with a deep scratch, it skipped every other word. No matter what I tried, it would not work. I didn't want to touch it, for fear I would scratch it even more, so I simply began blowing air on it gently, imagining that the air delivered my love to the CD. I then put it in and it worked perfectly, not skipping a single word.

When you recycle objects, you show your respect for the souls of things. When you throw things away that would not be useful to anyone else and release them with gratitude, you also become free. When you are generous with good things you no longer need and give them to others, you are inviting the Kingdom to be generous to you. When you have only what you need in the amounts that you need and stop hoarding or accumulating possessions, your mood and health will improve. If your house is overflowing with unloved things and your garage and shed are full of unwanted and untouched things and you have a storage unit where unopened boxes of things sit unexamined for years, your personal energy and life force is depleted. Free yourself and travel lightly through the world so that you can experience your days and nights fully. These are the laws of the Universe.

Love Your Few Good Things

I challenge you to walk around your house touching EVERYTHING you own with love; it will be quite eye-opening. Touch every single thing no matter how big or small. This includes the inside of your drawers and closets. And for the "advanced" readers, talk to every single thing you touch. Ask it if it is happy in your house, if it receives enough love from you, if it likes where it is placed, and if it needs cleaning or fixing.

You attach your personal energy to everything you own. It's not a choice, it's a law of the Universe. Everything you own affects you in either a positive or a negative way. The fewer possessions you have, the *more energy* you have. Gypsies have always had very few possessions. All possessions of a Gypsy family fit into a wagon. This gives us good health and a long life. Roma say, "If a journey is long, you can't take much along."

Romanies began moving into houses only in the past hundred years. If a family could choose how they wanted to build the house, it would have just one big room (even if there were ten family members). In the beginning, there would be no furniture except a low table. Everyone would sleep on the floor on feather mattresses near each other for the companionship of being together during sleep. Everyone would eat at the low table by sitting on the floor. Later, Romani families began adding a little bit more furniture and other things, but each would be carefully selected and carefully placed with great care in just the right spot. The house would be so clean that no one would be able to find a spot of dust in any corner.

When I got married, my family lived in a Romani way – one big room with mattresses on the floor and minimal furniture – but five years later we decided to buy a house. We selected our house in an unusual way. I would stop the car next to a house, walk around it, listen, and feel. Romanies take our surroundings very seriously. After all, you have to be able to understand where it is safe to stay overnight when you are constantly traveling from town to town. When I found the place I liked, I walked through the front door, hurried through the house, and walked outside through the back door. The backyard is the biggest "room" of the house, and the most important to me. I saw lots of trees, bushes, flowers, and rocks. The birds were singing, the butterflies soaring, and the energy of the place felt wonderful. I decided to buy the house without even looking at the rooms inside because I could tell we would be happy there.

The first thing I did was to get to know the house Guardian. Romanies and Russians believe each house has a Guardian. The Guardian does not protect the people living in the house, but rather protects the spirit of the house. If people don't take care of the house, don't love it, and don't keep it clean, the Guardian gets mad and plays tricks on the inhabitants. He can start by making them lose things and eventually end up making them sick. If the inhabitants express their love for the house and take good care of it (or better yet, recognize and respect the Guardian), the Guardian shows appreciation by keeping them healthy and relaxed inside their home. The Romani word for the house Guardian is Kharitko (from kher, meaning *house*) and the Russian word is Domovoj (from dom, also meaning *house*).

I made an intention to meet the Kharitko of my home during my sleep. What I did not expect was to see a nightmare. In the dream I saw a very scary looking woman (typically Kharitko is a man), with an angry face and extremely long nails. She said we were not welcome in the house and threatened to get rid of us. I woke up with my heart pounding. During the day I talked to the neighbors and found out that the previous owner had died in the home from cancer. His misery had created things we would have to deal with in order to live there happily. There was a lot of work to be done to turn Kharitki to our side. Luckily, I knew exactly what to do.

I started by cleaning the entire house; I paid attention to every inch of space, including the walls, ceiling, carpet, doors, and windows. As I cleaned the walls, I stroked them with love. I spread sea salt around the house and left it there for the next twenty-four hours to absorb the negative energy. Then I swept it all away while singing joyful songs. I opened all the windows and went around the house clapping my hands, moving the negative energy out of the windows and inviting positive energy in through the doors.

After the house was clean in body and spirit, it was time to fill it with beautiful music, songs, laughter, lovely things, and an abundance of fresh food. I even left some food for Kharitki as a sign of good will. After some time passed, I saw Kharitki in my dream again. This time it appeared as a kind old woman, her face soft with wrinkles and her eyes sparkling with mischief. She said that she and the Fairies of the garden had a chat and that they'd like us to plant berries and flowers. She also mentioned that she liked bread with honey and berry jam. I did what she and the Fairies requested, and the fresh berries in the garden abounded, and a little honey and jam on good Russian bread was left out from time to time.

Where Things Belong

Romanies have very strict rules about the art of placing things in the house. The most precious things have to be placed high from the floor. The floor is considered energetically unclean and because of that, it has to be spotless. We don't put things there, never a plate or a dish or a handbag. Dishes are highly regarded and placed high up on the shelves. Mirrors hold a lot of power and have to be kept very clean. Each room has to have a lot of open space in the middle so that the energy is not trapped by furniture and things. Romanies say, "We need the air." A table is placed in the middle of the room only during a celebration to accommodate a lot of guests. It is then moved back to the wall to allow the energy of the home to circulate.

I place the furniture and everything in my house with an intention. I focus on what I want to happen in my life, completely detached from the end result. I am in love with the process and I always have so much fun! The success of this way of keeping a house is head-spinning. As soon as everything was perfect, I instantly found the job of my dreams and my health and happiness soared.

The most amazing part was that when I applied the Romani art of placement to my friends' houses, they too had breathtaking results. One of my friends asked me to help her fall in love. I made some changes to her apartment and a few weeks later she had a wonderful boyfriend. One night, she called me with a plea: she only wanted one man, but so many men were attracted to her that she didn't know how to handle the pressure and wanted me to lessen the energy of attracting men, which was now so present in her apartment. The results are different for different people. My results were breathtaking because I did the art of placement with a Gypsy twist and put all of my love behind it. My thoughts played an important role in creating the change. The art of placement, just like any other ritual, is opened as a gate into what many call "being in the flow," or "in the zone," which is a creative place in the Universe where thoughts become reality.

To live well in my home, I talk to all the things inside my house, asking them to help me enjoy life. Gypsies think it is perfectly normal to talk to your pillow or your cup. One time, my favorite cup slipped out of my hands. Our kitchen floor is covered with tile and the cup would surely break. But in a split second I was able to shout, "Don't!" before the cup hit the floor. It heard me, protected itself, and didn't break. It didn't even chip. When I place a certain object in a certain area, I ask this object to help me make my wishes come true. I also became friends with Kharitki. This is why my results at home were so great.

Talk to your house and everything in it. Furniture and other items made from wood keep a memory of the place where the tree grew up, of the people who cut it and created things out of it. All things absorb your emotions and thoughts over time. Swearing at the things you own, calling them bad names, slamming doors, hitting or throwing things may not damage them physically, but will definitely damage their energy field. And instead of working for you, they will begin working against you because they are not aligned with good energy.

I am a Gypsy and we speak plainly. I say direct things but with a big smile. Imagine me standing in front of you reaching out with loving arms and say these things insistently and from my heart. There is no way you can have a happy, healthy, and successful life in clutter, uncleanliness, disorder, and ugliness. If you are living with any element of these things in your home, office, or car, you must turn this around as quickly as you can. If you are accustomed to living in this unhealthy way, then you must find examples of how you can live differently and create a vision and a plan for how you will live in health and beauty. Ask for emotional support from your taboro to increase your energy so that you will no longer tolerate clutter, dirt, and ugliness.

Once your vibration is raised, you will not put up with treating yourself and your precious life with disrespect. You were meant to experience order, cleanliness, and beauty in your life— in how you dress and in everything you touch. You are worth it! Beauty is your birthright. You are meant to live fully before you die, and I will be part of your support to get there. Who else do you know who can help? If you need extra help from an expert to help you clear the clutter, hire them and sell whatever you need to in order to pay them if you can't immediately find the money. The only *things* that have any value in this life are the things that support a healthy life. Everything else is a burden. Free yourself from your burdens—now!

Problem: You have too much stuff that you don't love and don't use.
Solution: Have a yard sale, give away things in good condition to friends and relatives, donate, recycle, and finally throw away things that cannot be used or recycled.

Problem: You are too attached to stuff.

Solution: Thank each thing for serving you. Take a picture of it if you'd like. Decide which things you really care about, frequently use, and love. Leave only the things you can't live without. Roma are not attached to any possessions, even essential ones. Everything we own is frequently exchanged. Things benefit from movement just as much as you do. When someone passes away in a Romani family, all possessions of this person are burnt. In modern times, they are given away or sold to gadje (non-Romanies). And yes, I mean *all* possessions, including all personal items, the car, and even the house. The only things that matter are the memories.

Maybe you have heard, but maybe you have not, that things have souls. Things know everything about themselves; more than you know about them. A beautiful thing is proud of itself; it likes to show off, spreading joyful energy around itself and helping you. A thing that is not beautiful or is broken is shy; it tries to shrink, pulling its positive energy in, spreading out sad energy. If you use something often and with love, speak well of it, and then watch as it starts to glow, like the Sun. But if you don't use something for a long time and it is neglected, it gets upset; as it begins crying, it spreads suffering and damage to the space around it. Better have few things that you truly love. Things that are your favorites appreciate being used often and with affection. Think about your things the way you think about pets: keep them clean, pay attention to each of them, feed them with your love. And if you don't love or don't use them, give them to someone who will appreciate them. There is always someone who will accept what you offer with great joy. Someone is dreaming about this thing they desire, yet it is dying away in your house. Let it go to the place it will be loved. Surround yourself with things you love and use, and they will surround your home with energy of joy, health, and wealth of the most meaningful kind.

Happiness is Free; Gratitude is Priceless

If you ever look at pictures of Romanies who live in very poor conditions, such as make-shift plastic tents with all of their possessions fitting into one meager bag, you will notice joyful, bright smiles. How can someone who has almost nothing be so happy? This is because they are grateful for what they have: their life, their family, and their taboro. These are the best things.

Be grateful! Be grateful for everything in your life. Thank everyone in your life. Thank God for you being alive or thank your parents. Thank water for cleansing you. Thank birds for their lovely songs. Thank your body for serving you so well. Thank flowers for their beauty. Thank mountains for their magnificence. Thank all people that you meet during your life, all people, without exceptions! Thank our Earth, thank the Sky and the Sun. Thank oceans, rivers, and streams. Thank your family members, friends, and co-workers every day. Thank your pets. Thank your house. Thank every individual thing in your house. The entire Universe was created for you to experience happiness. And the entire Universe deserves your gratitude.

I feel enormous gratitude for being lucky enough to see, to hear, to speak, to walk. So many people don't have these abilities. Thirty-seven million people in the world are blind. Did you know that? Have you ever appreciated your ability to see? The first thought that comes to my mind when I wake up—and open my eyes that can see—is deep gratitude. I constantly feel gratitude and love towards everything that surrounds me. When I wake up, I enter the magical feeling of happiness, a feeling that celebrates life. "I wish all people were healthy, joyful, kind, and happy." I walk out of the house looking forward to a great day full of adventure and happiness. I know that the Universe will arrange to bring me the information and experiences that my soul needs at this time.

We are not separate from each other. We are not separate from the Earth. We are not separate from the Universe. The most important lesson in life is to learn to feel this connection in every moment. When you turn on the light, ask yourself – where does electricity come from and who can I thank for it? When you eat an apple, think about the person who picked this apple. When you buy clothes, think about the person who made the clothes. Thank everyone and everything and see how the world will change in front of your eyes.

Right now it is fashionable to say that you can "attract money" quickly. Just look at a few books in any bookstore. You may read all these books and still not get rich. But everyone can revive the rewarding relationship with the Earth and other parts of the Universe.

So many rich people are depressed and use drugs and alcohol because their spiritual connection with the Universe is broken. Even if you have very little, be grateful for whatever you have and don't forget to thank everyone in your life.

A Rom wanted to get rich quickly. He had heard stories about hidden treasures and decided to find one. He searched here and there but with no luck. One day, he was sitting next to the fire when an old man approached him. "Why are you so gloomy?" the old man asked.

"I've heard stories about hidden treasures, but they are all lies. I've searched everywhere and didn't find anything," responded the rom.

"I know where you can find one," said the old man. "You see, I am very old and don't have much time left to live. I'll show you where to find the treasure."

So they went deep into the forest. The old man showed the Rom a certain place next to a big rock and asked him to dig. The Rom dug and dug and suddenly his shovel made a sound. It was a small chest. The Rom opened the chest and it was filled with gold! Elated, the Rom ran home with the chest. He woke up his wife and whispered, "Look, I found treasure!" He opened the chest but it was filled with rocks. Shocked, he told the whole story to his wife. She grinned. "Did you thank the old man?" she asked.

Heart Has a Higher Price than Wealth

In the past, Gypsies would have only one meal a day – dinner. Gypsy women would prepare the food and share it with all members of the taboro. If some families didn't make any money during the day and had no food, they would still eat with everybody else.

Sharing is a very important concept for Romanies. Imagine making a meal and then going around your neighborhood knocking on the doors and saying, "Dinner is ready!" Gypsies share money this way as well. Can you imagine sharing your salary with your neighbors? If you did, wouldn't that make your neighborhood feel like a vibrant community—if you were all looking out for each other in that way?

Romanies visit each other without invitation. A guest is highly respected. If you come to my home, I will put on the table my very best dishes and get everything I have from the refrigerator and off the shelves to feed you. Gypsies are famous for their hospitality. The concept of sharing is taught to us from a very young age. If one family visits another family and the guest child favors a particular toy, be assured that this toy will be given to him as a gift.

The generosity is mutual. No guest will ever come empty-handed as well. Food for the table and gifts for the children are a must. My daughter was accustomed to this spirit of generosity and would bring her toys to school and give them away to her classmates. She stopped after she noticed that no one else was doing the same with her. It is harder to be generous when everyone else is taking you for granted, or only taking rather than giving as well. When I lived in a dorm in Russia, I would buy the dishwashing liquid for everyone and do the dishes left in the sink — piles and piles of dirty dishes. But when I left my plate in the sink one day and no one washed it, and when the tenth bottle of dishwashing liquid had run out and no one refilled it, my sense of generosity was diminished.

In far-off days, a peasant walked in the forest. He walked and walked and along the way he met an old man. The old man was dirty and hairy, his clothes were torn and shabby. "Help me, kind man, you see how poor I am, give me alms, please."

The peasant staggered back, "Who, me? I am poor too; I can barely make both ends meet. If I share with you, I will deprive myself." And with that the peasant walked away.

The next day, a Rom was walking the same path through the forest and also met the old man. "Help me, kind man, you see how poor I am, give me alms."

The Rom replies, "I am simply a poor Gypsy, I have no money, but I have some bread." With these words, the Rom pulled a piece of bread from his bag and split it in half. He gave one half to the old man. They sat on two stumps and ate the bread.

The old man said, "I have a way to thank you, Gypsy. The stump I am sitting on is not an ordinary stump. Beneath it there is buried treasure. I am old, feeble, and can't dig it out. You are young and strong, you will manage it."

The Rom took a thick branch, dug a bit around the stump, then grabbed the stump and began pulling. Pulling once, pulling twice, and finally he pulled the stump out on the third try. And deep in the earth, he saw a chest. He dragged it out, shook off the dirt, and opened it. Inside, he saw precious stones, jewelry, silver and gold coins. The Rom gasped and said, "Well, old man, here is your treasure." No one replied. The Rom looked around, but the old man had disappeared. Only then did the Rom realize that it wasn't an ordinary man he had fed, but the Father of the Forest, Veshitko Dad. The Rom lifted the chest on his shoulder and carried it to the taboro to share.

Really Belonging

One way of living is full of energy and feeling connected to others, and the other is isolated, self-involved, and ungenerous. Which way do you want to live?

Surround yourself with good people; help them and let them help you. Balance and harmony are maintained by mutually beneficial relationships, so find them and nurture them. Great friends are great wealth.

Once when I was young, my family visited a beautiful beach that was littered with trash. We began to pick up the trash while everyone else was basking in the Sun. It quickly became obvious that we could not do it all by ourselves. Life would be so much easier if everyone cared. But we did what we could that day and I will always remember that beautiful day and what I had learned.

The winters in Russia are very cold. Gypsies could not travel during the winter. They would come to a village and ask the villagers if they could stay in their houses. For hundreds of years, villagers, especially poor ones, would agree. But during the last century, things changed. During one hard winter, a taboro was going from village to village asking for a place to stay. All of the villagers refused. The nights were getting colder and colder and the taboro still had no place to stay. During the night, a blizzard swept through the place where the taboro had set up their tents. The whole taboro froze to death. All the men, all the women, all the children, all the babies, all the animals. Can you imagine what it was like for the villagers who had not allowed them shelter to face the consequences of what they had done?

When I think of this story, I pay attention to the consequences of my actions. We do not live in isolation. An act of kindness or the absence of an act of kindness may have a much larger impact than we can possibly imagine. We are writing the history of our cities, towns, and neighborhoods today by our actions. We will either be there for each other or turn away. We have the opportunity to change lives for better or worse by choosing well. We are all tied together. Let's make our world a better place to live.

Romanies have very kind hearts. Thinking about others comes before thinking about oneself. We know we belong. We know that if we are good to each other, we will all thrive. Stinginess is ridiculed;

generosity is praised. "A stingy man has only a stomach, but a kind man has a heart."

Kindness in Action

Some major shifts happen in your life when you start being kind to yourself, kind to others, kind to other people's children, kind to animals, and kind to the Earth. And this is Gypsy wisdom—be kind even to the people you don't like. Anger decreases your energy while kindness increases it. The Universe understands and helps you when you feel the emotion of love. Unconditional love. If you imagine their point of view as if you were inside their minds, you can find a positive side to people that you might not have seen otherwise. The world will mirror your thoughts. What you wish for others will come back to you. This is why Roma say, "Whatever you do, good or bad, you will do to yourself."

Stay Calm in the Storm

Unhappy people are contagious and behave in ways that make others around them unhappy too. I once watched a woman storm into a gas station, rudely cut ahead of others in line, be rude to the person at the register and then, when the screen asked her to rate her experience, she hit the "bad experience" answer and stormed out. We all stood there speechless. If someone is rude to you, your first reaction may be to be rude back to them. It takes a lot of practice and mastery to stay calm when someone is screaming at you. When you see unhappy people, imagine good things happening to them. Don't wish bad things for people who behave in a way you find inappropriate. If you are happy, help others become happy too. Share your happiness any way you can: by smiling, saying encouraging words, giving help, or simply by giving a hug. I noticed that Americans don't hug very often, yet a big hug from the heart is a wonderful way to create happiness anywhere you go. A hug erases the distance between people and makes us kinder to each other.

When you are sick, wish for all people to become healthy. When I had headaches, I used to say, "May all people be free from headaches and the causes of headaches." When you are sad, wish for all people to become happy. We are all interconnected. It is extremely difficult to be a happy person if everyone else around you is unhappy, but this effort will return to you manifold. My daughter starts singing a silly song if I've had a hard day at work. I can't help but smile, and our evening is kinder and more loving.

Share your money, share your things, share your time. I donate to the organizations that help protect the wilderness and share my clothes with the homeless. I am constantly giving things away. I enjoy shopping for others more than I enjoy shopping for myself. When you share everything with joy, the Universe finds multiple ways to reward you. A giving hand will never be empty.

Problem: You feel miserable.
Solution: Find someone who is in a much worse situation than you are. This may be a homeless or chronically sick person, a disabled or abused child, or maybe even a whole Romani village, living at the edge of poverty and discrimination. There are millions of people who are in a much, much worse situation than you are. Give them a hand and you will realize that your life is not misery at all; it is a blessing.

One day a peasant was riding in a cart from his village to a remote town. He got tired and decided to take a nap. A Gypsy was passing by and saw the peasant sleeping on the grass and the cart with a horse nearby. He decided to play a joke on the peasant. He quietly led the horse to the forest and tied it to a tree. Then he came back and put the harness on. He began to neigh and stomp his feet like a horse. The peasant woke up, realized that his horse had disappeared, and began asking, "Where is my horse? What have you done with my horse?" The Gypsy responded, "I am your horse. A witch turned me into a horse five years ago. She told me that I would be a horse for five years and then turn back into a man. The five years are up today." At this point the Gypsy pulled some grass, put it into his mouth and spit it out saying, "I can finally eat some real food!" The peasant listened quietly and then said, "How will you buy the food? You don't have any money! Here!" and he gave the Gypsy most of his money. The Gypsy took the money and slowly walked away. He was thinking about the peasant and his kindness. He returned the horse to the peasant along with the money and said, "Kind peasant, please forgive me, I wanted to play a joke on you, but you taught me a good lesson. I will tell you how to find my taboro. And if you ever need help, you can always count on me."

Ten

Turning to the Higher Power

In Our Dreams We Fly to the Sun

A Rom experienced the same dream every night. In the dream, he walked in the forest among tall green trees carrying a shovel. He stopped next to a birch tree, dug a big hole, and in the hole there was a chest. He pulled it out, opened it, and found gold. Every time the Rom awakened from this exciting dream, he grabbed a shovel and went to the forest. He walked and walked, only there are many birches in the forest. Which tree was the one? After much thinking, the Rom made up his mind: I need to mark this birch in my dream; a red ribbon will do.

The next evening, the Rom found a red ribbon and before he fell asleep, he clasped it tightly in his fist. He had the same dream: he walked with a shovel in the forest, stopped next to a birch tree, and started to dig. At this very moment the red ribbon fell out of his hand. He picked it up and tied it on one of the branches. Then he dug up the chest and woke up. So the Rom jumps to his feet and   he can't find the ribbon. He grabs a shovel and runs to the forest. He walks here and there and looks there is a birch with a red ribbon on one of its branches! The Rom begins digging next to the birch. Digging and digging and then the sharp sound ding   the shovel hits something hard. He pulls a chest, opens it, and there what do you think there is?

I always fluff my pillow before I go to bed; I fluff it gently, as if the pillow were alive; I don't use force and I never beat it up. I lay my head on the pillow and it sinks into softness and lightness. This is my favorite moment – to immerse myself in the mysterious depths of the pillow, to shift my consciousness from reality to fantasy. And the pillow, the guardian of dreams, slowly opens a gate to the Otherworld.

I lay my head on my magical pillow, the one I have used for so many years, the one that holds so many of my good dreams, close my eyes, and think about my great-grandmother. She was a Gypsy fortune-teller. She could see the future as well as you can see this page. She had three daughters, but my great-grandpa wanted a son. My great-grandma told him that she could give him a son, but it would cost her life to do so. He insisted. She gave birth to a baby boy Mihail, my future grandpa, and then she died. It was 1913. In 1914 my great-grandpa was called into military service in World War I. He was soon killed and my grandpa was raised by a Gypsy taboro.

My pillow is very old. I've had it since I was a little girl. No one remembers where it came from, but I like to think that it once belonged to my great-grandma. At least that would explain why my pillow knows the future. She was known to have great powers of sight. Once in a while I see a dream that shows the events exactly the way they will soon happen.

My co-worker was only twenty-five weeks pregnant when I saw a dream that she delivered two tiny babies. When I came to work, I was relieved to see her office door open, but an hour later she told me she began having contractions and left. A few hours later she delivered her twins prematurely.

I have learned to distinguish dreams that have important messages from those that have insignificant ones. When I wake up after seeing a meaningful dream, I feel an urge to write it down immediately. I literally jump out of bed and grab a piece of paper and a pen. Trivial dreams do not leave an imprint in my mind, and usually there are no emotions attached to them.

In one of the special dreams, I saw myself inside a small spiritual bookstore. There were shelves with books written in English and Russian. There were also tables with jewelry and crystals. Wind chimes were hanging from the ceiling. Beautiful paintings hung on the walls. It felt so good to be inside this little bookstore. I looked around as a gentleman walked in and approached the cashier. He said, "I am looking for books by Natalia Kovaleva." I didn't hear what the cashier replied; I was thinking about the name "Natalia

Kovaleva." I've never heard of this author before. This is when I woke up. I wrote the name down on a piece of paper and went to work.

I decided to check if an author with this name existed in the database of Russian books on the Internet. I entered "Kovaleva" in the search window. In a few seconds I got the result. The first shock came when I realized that this author did exist – N. Kovaleva. The second shock and delight – when I read the description of her books: she writes about what happens to people when they dream! Of course I immediately purchased her books and studied them. They were fascinating and have made a big contribution to my life and work.

Sometimes I receive messages for my friends and relatives while I dream. One night, I saw my cousin. She was wearing very beautiful clothes and I asked her, "Where did you get these beautiful clothes?"

She replied, "Africa."

I asked her, "Is this the name of the store?"

She replied, "No, they are from Africa." My cousin had never mentioned anything about Africa to me, so I was puzzled. When I woke up, I wrote the name of my cousin on a piece of paper and "Africa" right next to it. I turned on my computer and typed my cousin's name and the word "Africa" into Google. The results I got were even more puzzling. Here is what I read: "Part of the beauty of the work of Malidoma and Echoes of the Ancestors is to see the flowering of the divinational healing arts in the West. To be a diviner is to be a healer…The following is a list of Dagara-style trained diviners." Then, there was my cousin's name! Because I did not even understand half of the words, I decided to call my cousin. She picked up the phone and I asked her, "So, what is it about you and Africa?" She was speechless. She did not tell anyone about her interest in Africa. After I told her about my dream, she confessed: she wanted to adopt a baby from Africa but was keeping it secret. She was afraid her family would be against this decision. My dream gave her the support she needed because she saw how our lives were linked and felt that her desire for a child in these particular circumstances was aligned with the purpose of her life, destiny, and wishes. Several years later, Malidoma, the shaman from Africa, was visiting my town and I had a chance to meet him. He told me I'd write a book and that it would be very successful.

In my dreams, I also communicate with my ancestors. Ancestors are extremely important in Romani culture. They provide guidance and answer questions in the most compelling and challenging situations. Your ancestors are always willing to be your teachers if you reach out to them and ask.

In one of my dreams I saw myself in my old apartment in Estonia. I knew that very wise men, healers and sages, holders of esoteric knowledge, were gathered in the guest room. The door to the guest room was half-open and I decided to walk in after some hesitation. I saw my father among the guests. I was surprised to see him there. He had passed away some time ago. I asked him how it was possible. He grinned.

"After we die, we go into transformation. It is similar to a dream state," he said. "Look at your body; is it your body?" Of course it is! I had no doubts about that. "The truth is, your physical body is asleep on your bed, under a blanket, but this does not prevent you from feeling your 'mental body,' just like your physical one. You can see it, move your arms and legs, talk, wear clothes, and you can communicate with me. This is as real as physical matter, except it consists of mental matter."

I was in shock. First of all, until that point I did not know I was dreaming. Second, it was the first time I had seen my physical body looking lifeless but asleep on my bed. It was a bit frightening, but fascination took over my fear, and I could see that I was not waking up. We continued our conversation. I said that I would like to learn more about mental bodies and our hidden abilities to use them, but I was not sure if anyone would be willing to teach me. At that time, one of the most impressive sages in the room got up and said that the education in his school took forty years but that he would teach me, for example, how to remove any pain with just my hand. "That long?" I asked, and immediately woke up. I was disappointed with myself. I could have said "Yes" right away! Teach me! Does it matter how long the education is? The process of education gives us new knowledge, and this process may go on for as long as we live. "I am so sorry," I shouted in my awakened state. "I accept, please take me in!"

My plea was heard. I even received several teachers, and with the teachers, I received lessons, tests, and exams as I dreamed. Some parts of this book are the result of what I learned. Others I am saving for later.

SWEET DREAMS EXERCISE

Before you go to bed, fluff your pillow gently. Ask for its help in sending you wonderful dreams. When you wake up, try to remember your dreams. What happened during your dreams? How did they make you feel? Love your pillows, take good care of your pillows, dress them in cotton and silk, and most importantly, cherish them. They will respond to your care by giving you the most wonderful dreams, and who knows, maybe one of them will even start predicting your future, become a bridge between you and your ancestors, or provide a school for you to learn something you've always wanted to know as you dream.

Problem: You have nightmares.
Solution: What you see in your dreams is a reflection of your spiritual balance, or lack of it. When you are in harmony with the entire

world, your dreams are peaceful and sweet. Before going to sleep, try to clear your mental and spiritual energy of any negativity and allow a positive sense of calm and relaxation to fill you up. Fall asleep thinking positive thoughts and feeling in tune with the creative energies of the Universe, and sweet dreams will follow.

Give a Gypsy Woman a Plate and She Will Tell Your Fortune

A king heard of a Gypsy fortune-teller who lived in his kingdom. Whatever she predicted, it all came true. Oh, how he burned with desire to find out about his future. He sent his servants to search for the fortune-teller and bring her to the castle. Several days passed and the servants came back with the Gypsy. She was barefoot, her clothes were old and torn, but her eyes were shining with a mischievous sparkle. The king was sitting high on his throne. He glanced at her with contempt and said, "Well, go ahead, tell me what is waiting for me in the future." The Gypsy got out her tattered cards. "No, no," the king stopped her, "I don't believe in cards. Do you know any other way?"

The Gypsy said, "I can tell your fortune by your hand."

"What? To let you, a dirty beggar, touch my royal hand? Never!" During that time, the servants announced that the dinner was served. The Gypsy smiled, "I can use a plate." A plate? The king ordered his servants to bring the Gypsy a plate. Said-and-done.

The Gypsy took the plate, turned it with her hands this way and that way, and said, "In a year, you'll have a son and I'll have a daughter. Eighteen years will pass and your son will meet my daughter. He will fall in love with her at first sight and marry her."

Having heard these words, the king jumped off his throne, ran to the Gypsy, grabbed the plate out of her hands, and smashed it on the floor. "This will never happen, deceitful woman! Take her to the dungeon!" The soldiers grabbed the poor woman and locked her in a cell.

The next day, the guard brought some food to the Gypsy. He was intrigued by the woman. "Gypsy, is it true that you are a good fortune-teller?"

"Truth, the simple truth."

"What is waiting for me in the future; will you tell me?" The Gypsy finished her food, turned the plate over in her hands this way and that way, and said, "This night you will go into the forest. Take a shovel with you. You will walk not an hour, not two, but keep moving, and when you stop, you'll dig a hole next to a big oak. You'll find treasure there, pure gold. You will get rich, richer than the king!"

"Richer than the king?" The guard's eyes burned with greed. "How will I know when and where to dig?"

"I will help you."

The night came. The guard opened the cell, grabbed a shovel, and he and the Gypsy walked into the forest. They walked not an hour, not two, with the Gypsy showing the way. Finally, they saw a big oak. "This is it," said the Gypsy, "just like the one I saw. Dig here." The guard began to dig.

Ding! The shovel hit something hard. "This is treasure, this is wealth," said the guard." "I will buy a castle, golden cart, I'll have a crowd of servants, and they will follow my every whim." The guard pulled up something heavy. But it turned out to be a big rock. "Hey, Gypsy, where is the treasure?" But the Gypsy had vanished into thin air.

A year passed and the king had a son. The king knew that the Gypsy had run out of the dungeon, so he issued

an order to kill all Gypsy girls. In horror, the Gypsy taboro hid deep in a forest far away from the castle.

Eighteen years passed. The prince, the heir to the
throne, was hunting in a forest far away from the castle,
and as his hounds chased a fox as he followed them on a
horse. The prince lost his way. He wandered in the forest all day and finally saw smoke coming from a fire. He
approached the fire and saw a Gypsy taboro. A beautiful Gypsy girl was serving the tea. He had never seen
anyone more beautiful than this Gypsy girl. He fell in
love with her at first sight. He jumped off his horse and
greeted the Gypsies.

"I am the prince, the heir to the throne. Tell me, who
is the father of this beautiful girl and what is her name?"

One of the Gypsies answered proudly, "I am her father and her name is Rada. Why do you ask?"

"I have never seen anyone more beautiful than your
daughter. I would like to marry her."

Having heard these words, one of the Gypsy women
smiled. The father agreed. The whole taboro accompa-
nied the prince to the castle. The prince took the Gypsy
girl straight to his father.

"This is Rada," he said, "she will be my wife." As
soon as the king saw the Gypsy girl, his face turned

bright red from rage; he gasped for air and fell on the floor, dead.

Some time passed and a wedding was celebrated. Gypsies danced and sang with all their hearts. And what beautiful plates there were on the tables! If I would have been there, I would have told the fortune of all the gadje in the castle on that happy day.

Every year my workplace holds an employee appreciation day. Free pizza gathers a big crowd. Yet for those who consider themselves motivated by intellectual things and would not be attracted by pizza alone, they throw in a free book to serve as bait. This year the organizers invited fortune-tellers and palm readers to lure even more people to have fun together.

I went to get a book. The bookstand had attracted a lot of people. I couldn't even see the books behind the human wall. I acted with faith and fun and squeezed my arm between the bodies to grab a random book, knowing it would be perfect. When I pulled the book out and looked at the cover, it read, *There Are No Accidents*. Of course. I have yet to meet a person who has more happy "coincidences" than I do. Nothing else interested me, so I connected with my colleagues and returned to the office.

One of my co-workers, Nora, is someone I didn't know well but knew that she called herself an atheist. She was intrigued by fortune-tellers and palm readers. As soon as I saw Nora, I asked her if she knew her future, if she had become acquainted with her destiny. She said that the line to see a fortune-teller or a palm reader was so long that she didn't want to wait. She asked me to tell her fortune, but I wasn't sure if she could set aside her belief about not believing. I said that I prefer reading auras. Nora asked me to read her aura right away. I declined at first because these gifts must be treated with respect, and if she saw this as a novelty there would not be the proper level of honoring us both. These are not parlor tricks. I wasn't sure if she was ready. Nora insisted. I finally agreed.

I needed several minutes to shift my consciousness from work to the calm state of mind necessary for a reading. I asked Nora to stand against a white wall in a co-worker's cubicle and I unfocused my eyes. In a minute I saw her aura. Nora was impatient, "What, what color is it?" I said, "It's lime green with some yellow sparkles here and there."

"What does that mean?"

"By my interpretation, what I'm seeing means that you are healthy, yet you are frequently concerned about your health. You have a very peaceful personality; you are friendly and expressive; you don't need much in order to be happy. Yellow sparkles mean to me that you have a wonderful sense of humor and are very intelligent, yet you tend to doubt yourself."

Nora was impressed. "You've got me all figured out," she said. I explained that it was the gift I developed and not me.

The next day I saw another co-worker, Laura. As soon as Laura saw me she shouted across the hall, "Read my aura, read my aura!" Obviously, Nora had told her. I declined. Some people think of these healing arts as some type of game. But I can tell a lot about a person by looking at the aura, and this can guide their future health and well-being. I can see if the person is angry, or sick, or even has a terminal illness. Most people are not prepared to hear bad readings and will get upset with the messenger. Laura pleaded to have a reading and would not take no for an answer. I agreed, thinking this would be the last time I'd do it in the office.

I asked Laura to stand against the white wall in the same cubicle and unfocused my eyes. The color of her aura was orange, but it also had "spikes" of energy going in all directions. I said, "You are very independent in your thinking; you are always busy, you always create plans for the future and work on several projects at the same time; you don't let other people do things for you. The 'spikes' of energy mean that you always give, give, give. You need to slow down, focus on yourself, and receive energy from others. Take time to create what *you* want in life, to pursue *your* passion."

"Yes," Laura said. "This is so true. I always had a feeling that I don't ask for anything for myself, but I've never done anything about it. Thank you!"

It was Friday night, the last minutes of the working day, when suddenly my boss stepped into my office. "You must read my aura," he said. I saw Laura standing behind him. I could not believe she told him. No, no, no! I did not want to read Bryan's aura. I firmly refused. If I saw something bad, how would I be able to tell him? My intuition protested. I begged Bryan not to read his aura, but he would not leave. I gave in. I asked Bryan to stand against the white wall in the same cubicle and to close his eyes. I unfocused my vision and looked at his aura. Soon tears were running down my cheeks. The color of his aura was light brown. It meant that a disease had already started its destructive path through his body. I could tell that several years ago his aura had been the sunny color yellow. He had once enjoyed life to the fullest, but something had happened. I was certain he had stopped having fun. Anxiety and depression had replaced happiness and joy. I had never known the "sunny" Bryan. But I knew that if he continued to do what he was doing, this disease would become cancer, severe depression, or some other chronic illness.

I was able to control myself and quietly wiped away the tears. I was silent. Bryan was standing against the wall, his eyes closed. Laura was standing behind my back, waiting. What was I supposed to tell him now? Tell the truth and upset him? I am not a doctor and don't have the right to diagnose anyone. Not tell? And let my conscience torture me during the nights? I decided to tell the truth, but very carefully and gently. "Bryan, I can see that you used to have a yellow aura. You used to joke around and have lots of fun. But during the last several years, some emotional problems have begun to show up in your health. In order to take care of your health, you need to go back to that state of light-heartedness. Become the happy-go-lucky person you used to be. Start enjoying your life to the fullest. Otherwise it is possible that a disease will consume your body." Bryan responded, "You are right. Twelve years ago I saw life in a bright light. I liked being silly and laughed a lot. But during the last several years, I became too serious and worried. I would love to bring back this feeling of joy and fun." Bryan thanked me. Still, I think he was upset. During the next several days, I caught Bryan smiling to me and saying, "Back to yellow!"

Connecting As If By Magic

Long gone are the times when Gypsies traveled in wagons. Now we travel with a search engine as a tool for interacting with the Universe. Yes, the Internet is a part of the Universe too. I am so fascinated by it that I began writing my doctoral dissertation about it, "The Entropy of the Internet." There is nothing else in the entire Universe that connects us faster and easier. I use this information super-highway to receive instant messages from the Universe.

Try it. Think of a word, any word that has a special meaning to you. Now type it into a search engine and see what kinds of messages you receive.

Once I had a vision of a circle with a star on the edge. The feeling of this vision was magnificent and powerful. The circle looked like a full moon and the star seemed to be right on top of it. If I could paint, I would paint it right away and it would be an amazing piece of art. But I don't paint, and so instead I searched the Internet to see if a similar painting already existed. I was wondering how to go about that when the word "creativity" popped into my mind. So I typed "creativity" into Google and then just clicked and browsed, clicked and browsed. It took me some time, but the end result was so worth it! Finally, I saw a drawing done by an artist that had the circle and the stars, just like I had seen in my vision. There were several articles on the same web page that provided a missing link for my vision. Suddenly, it all made sense. I realized that we are all connected more deeply that we think, and the Internet lets us find this connection faster—as if by magic.

Wishes can be materialized so quickly with the technology we have at our fingertips today. I invite you to see the magic in what you can find and what shows up in your inbox as an unexpected email that, when you open, answers a wish. The way an app on your phone can open up worlds of possibility. How each new way to do something adds something special to your life.

I have a client who had a breakthrough in speaking her wishes and having them appear. I had been teaching her the need to cook fresh food, not overcooked, with beautiful colors, with high nutrition and a healthy and loving vibration. The problem was that she was very busy and didn't have the experience of loving to cook. I explained that working too hard was something that could undermine health and that stopping to cook would bring her great health, but she was adamant that she wasn't interested in cooking. The obstacles to cooking regularly were that when she wanted to make a particular dish and had a recipe, if she didn't have all the ingredients she would either make it anyway and miss key flavors, or she would have to take the time to run to the store for the few missing things. She was genuinely not interested in planning menus ahead of time, carefully shopping for all the ingredients, and organizing her life around cooking. It just wasn't her thing. It seemed we were stuck until, in her morning quiet time to create the magical intentions for the day, she dreamed up something as a powerful wish with the belief that this magical thing could come true.

She spoke into the world exactly what she wanted. This is what she invited into her life. Someone who was an innovative chef who had great ideas for making simple dishes that were easy to prepare, nutritious, and full of color and beauty would send her a box every week with the number of meals she wanted to cook this way. In the box would be everything she needed to make each dish, down to the lemon to zest and the fresh spices and herbs. She wished that the recipes would be beautifully designed on cards so that they would be a pleasure to prop up on the kitchen counter. There would be a photo of the finished dish and simple instructions she could follow while listening to music or watching the kinds of instructional video she liked to have fun with in the evening. Her request was for quick recipes that would empower her to love cooking and take care of herself in this simple, sensual way.

As soon as she completed her morning ritual, she sat down at the computer, and what was on her screen? An email from a company that provided the service she had just requested—down to the last detail. She knew that in order to invite more magic into her life, she had to honor the magic that showed up when she made requests like this, and so she immediately ordered the meals with gratitude and joy. They have delighted her for months now. Her health and well-being are very good. She is not intimidated by cooking. Her life is enhanced with this magic.

I had also asked her to drink several kinds of fresh healthy juice. She said she didn't have time to get the fresh produce and make the juice. Inspired by her previous success, she went to the Internet, put in the search terms, and in just a few minutes she had found the perfect juice, available daily, less than a mile away from her home. Ask and you will receive. It was all so perfectly what she had wished for, and now she is empowered to keep wishing for more of the experiences that will expand her health and prosperous life.

Your loving communication with the Kingdom has great power. The objects and images around you have power, your conversations have power, your requests of the Universe have power. When you bring reminders of the magic of life and what really matters to your surroundings, magic will happen every day.

I have a client who wanted to travel more, and so he placed his passport in a beautiful bowl on his desk with thoughtfully framed photos of places he wanted to go and the things he wanted to do. Suddenly, offers to work internationally started to arrive and friends started to suggest affordable getaways in new countries as group gatherings in beautiful private homes. There wasn't time to look for the best deals for airfare—but as soon as the request for magical help was made out loud, a friend called to suggest a personal assistant who worked by phone for a reasonable hourly rate and was a whiz with international travel. Your wish is the Universe's command, so invite this magic into your world by asking for what you want to receive.

Your Amulets and Charms

Amulets and charms are important. The easiest thing is to go into a beautiful place in nature with a prayer in your heart to find an amulet for protection or good luck. Go out, look around and decide in advance that you will come back from this magical hunting and gathering journey with something that has been magnetized to help you. Your eye will notice something, your hand will be drawn to pick something up. You will attract something unusual that is beautiful, symbolically important, a thing that speaks to you. You pick it up and hold it and it feels right. You say a chant or a prayer out loud to make it more powerful. "Let this object shield me, bring good luck, help me heal." And as you hold it in your hand you say these things and give it your attention and energy. Then take it home, and each time you need protection or good luck or health, you grab this object and let it reinforce your power. Carry it with you in your pocket or in little bag around your neck, or place it thoughtfully in a special place in your kitchen, office, porch, bedroom, or bathroom, depending on what you want. This sacred object will appreciate being called upon and will activate the energy needed to serve you.

Your movement through the world is important. Watch for and listen for wind and the feathers that are offered to you by the birds around you. The horseshoe is universally used for good luck and protection above doorways and needs to be upside down like the letter U in order to hold the luck. This is often still done throughout the Gypsy community. Anything that has to do with horses is considered good luck. Saddles worked with symbols are very sacred. Little horse statues can hold wonderful power.

The world is full of messages that are waiting for us. I always pay attention to the feeling that I have a message from the Universe waiting for me and I listen carefully. On a cold rainy day, things just seemed to fall apart. Because I do not believe in accidents, once something goes wrong, I start to wonder what it is I need to learn. I slow down to listen.

This time, I walked to a nearby café, got very cold and soaking wet, only to realize that I had forgotten my wallet. I walked back to work to grab my wallet and then returned to the café. Then my chiropractor's office called to reschedule my appointment for a much later time because the doctor had to attend a funeral.

I didn't want to wait for another reminder that there was a message waiting for me. After lunch, I began asking myself: What is the message? How do I get the message? I knew there was a message for me just as you know there is a message on your phone. The "accidents" or "breakdowns" are the blinking lights. So, how could I get the message? I sat in my office in front of the computer... And then I got a crazy idea to go to use Google and simply type "Message for Milana." I did that, and what a wonderful surprise! The first web site I bumped into was a site that provided valuable information about the very topics that were of most interest to me on that day. It was just the right time to connect with the information and people. As soon as I got the message, the problems in my day stopped. Thank you, Universe, for calling!

Speaking of technology, I'll never forget the first day years ago when I took my husband's cell phone with me. I had never used a cell phone before. I put it in my purse and forgot about it. Then I went to a bookstore and began browsing through the card section. I noticed a pretty Christmas card, picked it up, and opened it. At this very second, beautiful music began to play. Was the music coming from the card? I looked at the card from both sides, puzzled. It was a regular paper Christmas card with nothing hidden inside. No place to put a small battery. I closed the card. The music stopped. In a few seconds, I opened the card again and the same music began to play. It took me a while to realize that the sound was coming from the cell phone in my purse! I had experienced several moments of pure magic. It made my day. Don't you see, even approaching explainable things with a sense of magic can open up the world and provide delightful experiences when we choose to see the magic around us. A cell phone is a magical thing ringing in my purse, so even when I understood what was happening, I could be delighted that people had worked so hard to invent something as amazing as a cell phone. Pure magic!

CYBER-WONDER EXERCISE

Open a search engine. Think about your dreams and wishes. Type the first words that come to your mind. See what kind of websites appear. Listen to your intuition as you browse through the websites. You will be pleasantly surprised at what you will find.

Problem: You have an important question in mind and would like to use fortune-telling to find the answer.

Solution: Make tea using half a cup of loose tea leaves. Strain the tea and empty the leaves on a plate. Even out the leaves. Now focus on your heart and remember a happy event from your past. Smile, relax, and ask your question. Look at the tea leaves and unfocus your eyesight. Stare into the leaves on the plate and ask the question again. What is the first thing that comes to your mind? This is the answer to your question.

Problem: You tend to worry about your future.

Solution: Create your own Tarot cards. Take beautiful paper and cut it into rectangles the size of regular Tarot cards. Ideally, there should be 77 cards. Write a positive message on each card. For example, "Expect a happy event today." Or "You will have good luck tomorrow." Or "An amazing adventure is awaiting you." Or "You will enjoy great health." Each day shuffle the cards and pick up one card. Read the message several times. Say it out loud with a smile. Soon you will notice that these messages become true. We program our heart and mind by what we focus on, so dance with your own personal magic.

We Haven't Seen God but We Have Seen the Sun

One priest overheard that a Romani Shuvihano lived alone on a nearby island. By the by, people visited him from all over the world, and he cured many illnesses. "How was this possible?" asked the priest. Obviously, it needed to be explored. All right. The priest gathered some things and sailed to the island. He wandered around the forest for some time and finally found the Shuvihano. The Rom was sitting next to the fire, looking at the flames. The priest spoke, "Say, Gypsy, is it true that you can heal any person, cure any illness?" The Rom smiled and said, "Maybe that's true."

"How do you do that?"

"Simply," says the Rom, "I pray."

"But how do you pray?"

"I say, 'Oh Sun, our Father, oh Moon, our Mother, the Spirits of Fire, Air, Water, and Earth, heal this person, now!'"

"This is all wrong," said the priest in indignation. "I will teach you the right kind of prayer." And the priest taught the Rom the prayer from the Bible. Content, he set off home. As he was sailing back, he heard the

Rom's voice, "Wait, I forgot the words of the correct prayer." The priest turned his head and saw the Rom running fast over the water towards the boat, his feet barely touching the water. "Pray the way you always prayed," said the priest, "Don't change a word."

When you have to have something NOW, prayer is the best way to ask the Universe for help. There is a very powerful Russian movie about prayer called *Island*. It helped me learn how to pray. Once, my husband injured his fingers. A heavy metal plate fell on his hand. All of his nails were bruised blue but eventually grew back into health, all except one. The nail on his ring finger stopped growing. The blood collected under the nail and turned black. One month passed. At this time, a friend of mine gave me *Island* to watch. The main character of the movie prayed with such passion and such a strong belief that his prayer would be heard, that I got inspired. I prayed to get an answer about how to help my husband with his finger. I don't like the Russian word for prayer – *molitva*. It comes from the word meaning "to beg". Prayer is not a plea. It is not begging. It has nothing to do with fear or anger. Prayer is an offering of love. It is a pure emotion of sharing love from the bottom of one's heart. A prayer is a conversation with the Universe, with the force that has all the power in the world and all the love in the world. If a prayer can be answered, it will be. If it can't (for reasons we can't comprehend now—perhaps because what we want is not really right for us), no amount of begging will help. We are not inferior to the Universe, we are a part of it. All nations and tribes in the world, for thousands and thousands of years, have prayed to the different parts of nature. How would you talk to a mountain or to the Sun? Perhaps Alexander Pushkin, a Russian author who is considered to be the greatest Russian poet, will help.

Here is how he addressed the Sun:

"Sun, dear Sun! The whole year coursing
Through the sky, in springtime thawing
From the chill earth winter snow!
You observe us all below…"
The Moon:
"Moon, o Moon, my friend!" he said,
"Gold of horn and round of head,
From the darkest shadows rising,
With your eye the world apprising,
You whom stars with love regard
As you mount your nightly guard!.."
And the Wind:
"Wind, o Wind! Lord of the sky,
Herding flocks of clouds on high,
Stirring up the dark-blue ocean,
Setting all the air in motion,
Unafraid of anyone
Saving God in heaven alone!.."
(Translated by Peter Tempest).

If you are not comfortable talking to different parts of nature, would you at least talk to your own heart? If you feel love towards the whole Universe when you pray, your prayer will be heard. I always smile when I pray. I am talking to someone who cares deeply about me and is eager to help. It's a sacred conversation that leaves me with a feeling of gratitude and awe.

A prayer can be passionate, a prayer can be playful, a prayer is the expression of your creativity and can be a song, a dance, a whisper. When I pray, I always feel humble and grateful. I am so glad that I am not on my own when I face a difficult situation. Help from the entire Universe is always on its way.

So, what happened to my husband's finger as a result of my fervent and loving prayer? The next morning, a co-worker who had been on medical leave for some time suddenly called me. She was a nurse, so I asked her if she knew anything that would help a nail grow. She said she did! All I had to do was massage the finger from the base until the end of the nail several times during the day. I did that, and in a few days the nail began to grow. In a month, the old nail was gone, all blackness was gone, and I had learned to ask the Universe and those around me for answers, because we all collaborate together for our good.

Just remember that if your wish is not granted, the higher consciousness knows that it is not in your best interest. Don't force it and don't get discouraged. You will understand later why things turned out the way they did. Roma say, "Who asks God a lot, gets nothing." Trust the Universe. It is never wrong. We are never alone. The Higher Power is always right next to us—I encourage you not to forget that.

Problem: I am not religious. I don't believe that prayers are answered. **Solution:** Don't force yourself to believe anything. Romanies believe that the world around us is alive. Mountains are alive, the Moon is alive; animals, trees, and even inanimate things have a spirit. You don't have to believe that it is true. Simply *imagine* that it is true. *Pretend* that it is true. What would your life be like if the entire world around you was alive and listening to you? Who would you like to talk to? What would you like to ask?

Simply share your love with something you considered inanimate in the past and feel the energy of love returning back to you. If this something had all the power in the world and could help you in some way, how would you ask for help? Don't expect anything, just ask. Keep an open mind throughout this process, even if you can't accept it as truth. You will be surprised and delighted at what happens next.

A man was very poor. He had a tiny house where he lived with his wife and four children. He had to work day and night to support his family. He was never happy. One day he went to the desert a few miles from his village and began complaining out loud, "God, why did you forget me? Why do I have to work so hard and still remain so poor?" Suddenly, God appeared and said, "I will tell you, but first, bring me a glass of water; I am very thirsty." The man ran to his house, but something terrible had happened. It was a very hot summer and a wildfire had started. His house was burning. The man tried to put out the fire, but the house burned to the ground. It was a miracle that his wife and children were not hurt. Still, the man sat on the ground next to the burned house and cried out loud, "God, why me, why did you do this to me?" And then he heard the voice, "I'd like to tell you, but where is my glass of water?"

Take Your Happiness with Your Own Hands

An explosion on the Sun has impact on us; the phases of the Moon influence us; the birth of a new star is felt inside us. You can become aware of the interactions of energy between you and different parts of the Universe by tuning into these experiences. Ancient cultures knew all of this very well, but this energy exchange has been forgotten in most of the modern world. Whether or not you know it, energy exchange (between you and nature or between you and the man made world) happens every second. The energy of a place such as your home, your work space, a location in nature, each has an enormous influence on your body's energy and health and also on your emotional and spiritual health. A recent study showed that women who live surrounded by trees, plants and greenery were much healthier than those who didn't. To us Gypsies, that just makes common sense.

Our surroundings have much greater impact than what we are accustomed to thinking. Constant energy exchange between all living and artificial things and their surroundings happens every second. These energies have been described and engaged with for a very long time. Have you heard about Qigong? It is a series of energy exercises that originated in China. Surprisingly or not, depending on how you see the Universe, these exercises are very similar in essence to a Shuvihano's energy exercises.

This is my own interpretation of some historical facts. In Russian, the word "Gypsy" is translated as "tsygan" and Qigong is translated as "tsygun". These two words are pronounced almost identically, with the exception of just one vowel. The fact that these two words are pronounced almost the same is a "coincidence." Or is it?

Qigong appeared about four thousand years ago as a form of dance. At that time, people believed that being sick (physically, emotionally, or spiritually) was associated with the lack of energy movement. When people began performing Qigong (the energy dance), they would not only become healthy and experience peace, they would also start predicting the future with a higher sense of intuition. The development of intuition and an ability to predict the future is a very important part of Qigong. Qigong masters are healers and fortune-tellers. The goal of Qigong is to unite heaven, Earth and the human being. This resonates for me in many ways. The Romani flag depicts heaven, Earth, and the wheel that connects the two. This wheel is linked to the concept of chakras, the energy vortex of a human being (pointing to the Indian heritage of Gypsies). It is also known that Gypsies moved through China, the home of Qigong. I believe that the Gypsy dance is connected to the spontaneous dance exercise in Qigong. Whatever the source, this dancing with energy leads to spontaneous healing and the development of intuition. We are connected through history in our rich traditions. We are all one taboro.

Healing happens when the brain is not busy (and our brain is busy even during several hours of sleep). When you are looking at the clouds, letting your mind drift with them or meditating to quiet your mind, your brain doesn't have to process a huge amount of information and can focus on healing. However, if your mind is constantly busy, you are not allowing a key part of that healing to occur. If you don't have time to look at a leaf on a tree or to sit quietly and not think about anything, this is a sign that your life is out of balance. You have lost control. Your brain is no longer serving you if it is always active. You have become a slave instead of a creator.

My dream is that in my lifetime, or the lifetime of my daughter, some type of energy exercise will be practiced by every person on Earth, and so I am dedicating my life to bringing this healing to as many people as I can. Energy exercises have enormous healing power. I am surprised that not many people practice them. They are not necessarily controversial because they are not connected to any nationality or religion. The amazing art of healing the physical, emotional, and spiritual body (in record time and with unbelievable ease) is available to all. Anyone can do energy exercises: from very small children to 100-year-olds; from athletes to paralyzed people.

Qigong was a secret and so were Shuvihano's energy exercises, which were kept secret for about a thousand years. These exercises teach how to connect with the healing energy of the Earth and the Sky. By being between these two very powerful energy sources, a human being becomes a link that connects them and creates truly unlimited power. This power enables anyone to be in charge of his or her healing. Pretty impressive, right? It gives me enormous joy to have access to this ancient wisdom and to be able to share it openly. We live at a fortunate time.

Years ago, I learned Shuvihano's energy exercises from my parents. They divorced when I was very little. I was fortunate that my mother taught me how to access the healing power of Mother Earth and my father taught me how to access the healing power of Father Sky. It was the perfect way for me to learn and balance these energies. Because their teachings were separate, it took me a while to connect all the pieces.

I will never forget my first lesson with my father. I was a little girl and we were walking along a beautiful river under a night sky. There were hundreds of bright shining stars. It was so beautiful that I kept looking up. This is when my father said, "You know, you can bring the power of the stars inside you." And then he showed me the magic of the Universe. My father gave me the stars.

THE HEALING LIGHT AND EARTH MAGIC

On a night with no clouds, go to the best place to see stars. It is best if you can drive away from the city to avoid light pollution. Stand up straight and stretch your arms to the sides, palms up. Now look at the stars and bask in their healing light. Smile. Fill your body with the energy of the stars. This exercise seems very simple, but the results are profound.

My mother showed me how to connect with the Earth through bare feet and tempering the body with cold air and water. She also taught me about herbs and many other healing techniques.

Finally, when I connected the teachings of my father and mother, an amazing system of healing arose inside me. I realized these were the healing arts practiced for a thousand of years by Gypsy Shuvihanos. I just didn't know the name of the system that I was practicing. In the past, I wasn't consistent and did not perform the exercises every day. Then I received access to rare books and great teachers who were not well known. The Universe led me to key knowledge my father did not have the chance to pass on to me because I had been "too busy" with my life. After years of study it all finally clicked, just when I was ready to understand.

Shuvihano's energy exercises can only be practiced in places where the healing energy is high: your backyard will work if it's not located on a busy street. A great place to work with energy is an isolated beach, a park that is not crowded, or any beautiful remote spot in nature. These practices can only be done outside, as far as possible from man-made structures and noise. Being barefoot is best. If you are doing these exercises with a group of people, become acquainted with each other first and make sure that everyone has the same intention. Clear intention is very important in performing these exercises. If you have no other option but to perform these exercises at home and alone, please first make sure that your house is as clean as possible and keep the windows open at least thirty minutes before the exercises.

Many times, I perform Shuvihano's energy exercises on the beach. I first walk along the beach searching for a perfect place to do them based on how the place feels. It takes me a while, but finally I find an open space protected by little hills on three sides and the ocean right in front. The sand is the color of the Sun. I breathe with the ocean, exhaling when the waves crash and inhaling as they roll away from shore. The ocean is alive and gladly shares its powerful energy with me as I breathe with the rhythm of the waves.

When I visited Hawaii, for a while I thought I was the only one doing energy exercises on the beach. But one morning I came to my special power spot on the beach ... and found two men doing Tai Chi there. I felt enormous joy, as if I had gone to the Moon all by myself and suddenly found other people there. So, they kept doing Tai Chi and I did my energy exercises, silent energy dancers together with me on the fantastic beach, enjoying a special energy spot on the Earth.

PLUG INTO POWER DIRECTLY

This exercise must be done outside during the day. There should be no roof over your head. Don't do it if clouds obscure the sky. Stand up straight, extend your hands, palms down. Move them up and down in small movements as if you are flying. You will feel as if you have needles in your hands. Now bend your elbows in front of you. Open your palms. Your palms will face each other and the space between them should be a bit smaller than a volleyball. The fingers will be stretched out, a little bit backwards and apart from each other. You will feel a strong pulsation in the middle of your palms. Hold it for a few seconds. Now raise your arms up very quickly and with great force, as if you are trying to "plug in" to the sky. Lift your chin slightly, so that you can see the sky. Your whole body should be stretched up and held with power at the center. See the energy coming from the sky, through your arms, down to your body and into the Earth. Now feel the energy coming from the Earth into your bare feet, up your body, shooting into the sky. You have just connected the energy of the Sky with the energy of the Earth. Pay attention to every part of your body. Feel the power of the energy current.

Experiment by doing this exercise during different times of the day, during the sunrise and sunset. You will notice that the energy you receive will be quite different. The difference between this exercise and the next is your intention. "Plugging into Power" has the intention of receiving bright, bold, and powerful energy. The Cosmic Tree has the intention of receiving subtle, soft, calming energy.

THE COSMIC TREE

This is my favorite exercise for stress relief. Find a park or a beautiful place in nature. This exercise has to be done during the day. Take off your shoes and socks. Stand straight on the ground with your feet shoulder-width apart, your knees slightly bent. Softly "pet" the air with your hands. Now put your hands in front of your belly button, palms facing each other, shoulders relaxed. Close your eyes and imagine a warm current going between your palms. Soon you will be able to feel it. Your palms will start pulsating. Imagine that you are a tree. A big, tall, healthy tree. Your feet have roots. They go very deep into the ground. Through these roots, you are receiving healing energy of the Earth along with all the vitamins and minerals that you currently need. Feel very steady on your feet. Now imagine that the branches are growing out of your shoulders. They have beautiful, healthy green leaves. These leaves absorb the energy of the Sky, the Sun, and the Wind and pass it on to you. Try not to think about anything else. Just stand. Be the big tree. I can easily do this exercise for thirty minutes or more, but you might start slowly. Your intuition will tell you when to stop. We all have different experiences of time and you will know what is best for you. It's better to do this exercise a little bit at a time to get accustomed to it rather than not do it at all; try to spend at least ten minutes standing as the big tree connected to cosmic energy.

When my daughter was very young she saw me perform the Cosmic Tree exercise in our back yard many times. Finally, she asked if she could join me. I happily agreed. I explained the exercise to her, then closed my eyes and began transforming into a big healthy oak. I was sure she would run away after a minute of doing this exercise. How many little kids have you seen standing still for more than a minute? But when I opened my eyes twenty minutes later, she was still there, standing still with her eyes closed. "You can open your eyes now," I said. She opened her eyes and grinned. "I went to a magical world," she said. "It was so happy and peaceful there. I thought that my left hand was the Moon and my right hand was the Sun. Right after that I felt a magical door open and I thought, 'Home sweet home!' Even though it was the first time I experienced this place, I felt as if I missed this place so much! Everything seemed right and perfect. Then I began thinking about my favorite things. I imagined that these things were everywhere. Everything felt peaceful and relaxing. It started off as a thick, wild forest filled with many kinds of wild animals. Then it turned into a happy meadow with green, beautiful grass filled with many rabbits. After that it changed to a red, orange, and yellow canyon with lizards, birds, a few snakes, and more rabbits. Then it turned into the ocean with a sandy, warm beach, and the ocean was filled with fish and dolphins. Everything I loved was there–animals, plants, and sparkly colors. It is my magical world!" I was speechless. Kids never quite do what you expect them to do. They are capable of so much magic!

In the beginning it may be very difficult to "just stand' and "do nothing." We are conditioned by action movies and a noisy culture around us to expect something new every minute. When I watched Russian movies as a kid, often nothing would happen for several minutes. A man could sit on a porch looking at the rain, or walk along a street – just walk–with music playing and not much else happening for a few minutes. This gave the audience time to experience what he was experiencing.

The next time you watching a typical American movie, pay attention to the timeframes and action. You will notice that something happens EVERY SECOND! This provides little open space for the energy of storytelling to flow and for the experience of life to catch up with the audience.

My daughter once loved Russian cartoons and their nice relaxed pace with characters who could sit on a bench and think. Kids loved these cartoons because they left space for imagination and daydreaming. It was the difference between a blank piece of paper for drawing and coloring inside the lines of a coloring book, but after she began watching cartoons on American channels, she could not watch Russian cartoons anymore. Thank heavens she always kept the ability to connect with the natural world and enjoy the trees that call to both of us so powerfully.

Not Enough Nothing

We are over-stimulated by the wrong things. Our lives are crying out for grounding and simplification. We need to add more "nothing" to our lives. I see around me the constant evidence of how we now apply the action movie standards to our lives. We are accustomed to constant stimulation: TV, Internet, video games, conversations that don't have any real content, and music that is not thoughtfully chosen, but that is playing all around us. Everywhere we go we are being activated, supposedly entertained. Screens show us images and advertising and even restaurants have televisions hanging from the ceilings blaring content we don't invite into our lives. I see families at dinner together but there is no communication or connection—because each them is on a cell phone! There are gas pumps with screens broadcasting advertising and junk content. Everywhere. Too much of everything, not enough nothing!

We don't know how to just sit, walk in silence, connect with our loved ones, or do nothing and be perfectly content and at peace. The brain and body needs this quiet, this doing nothing, to heal and reflect and create.

It is during this time of nothingness and silence that the Universe talks to us. It is in these moments that the emptiness fills with magic. Learn to be slow and quiet at times so that you can communicate with the Universe and it can talk to you. If people have to pay for silence and pay for time to reflect by taking a class, we're adding commerce to things that are free and are doing so for no reason.

I imagine my Romani ancestors showing up and being shocked by our time. "They are charging you money for water! For clean air at an oxygen bar! And you pay to sit in silence to pray?!" It's hard to understand why we don't just make simple use of what is most important and be grateful for that simplicity.

The phrase "time is money" does not apply to Russians and Roma because life is life and is too precious to be bought and sold. People take several coffee breakes during the day because naturally you would stop to connect with others or just be quiet inside your own experience for a few minutes throughout the day. A Roma store would naturally close for lunch so that the people who work there could rest and eat together. And the whole country takes ten days off for the winter holiday break to do nothing. In Russia, the pace of life is slower than in the United States. Different cultures have different approaches to time. It's good to know these differences. In Russia, Greece, and Latin America, time is seen as an infinite resource. If your friends invite you to a party, you can be one hour late and no one will be upset because the party will start in waves as people arrive and leave. Russians use a famous proverb, "Those who are happy do not observe the time." And Roma say, "If you count every minute, you won't notice life," as well as "Don't count minutes and hours – better have fun."

Time is a strange concept. When I write, I am so motivated by love and my desire to share with people what I know that time speeds up. I am always shocked to find out that an hour has passed when I thought it was just five minutes of joy. Yet the first time I decided to fast for a day, time stopped. I thought the end of the day would never come. So now when I need extra time, I simply stop eating.

Tuning Into You

Because so many people run around watching the clock and not connecting to the natural world, it is helpful to slow down. This is a moment to "work" at playing with your energy and consciously feeling what you feel. Let's go into nothingness and give yourself a true break. Before you perform these exercises, you may want to learn how to feel energy with more sensitivity. Everyone is able to feel this energy. The way different people feel this energy is, well, different. I can only describe how I feel this energy and then see if you experience it similarly or differently. To me, the act of relaxing my body and mind feels as if someone is gently tickling me. Some people report feeling pins and needles, some say it feels like a warm current running through their body, but everyone agrees on one thing: it feels good! Why don't we do something that feels so good more often? Only because we don't think of it. Nut now we are, and I'm giving you permission to stop to feel your energy any time you want. You can make this demand of your life and everyone and everything in it. You get to stop and be with yourself!

Try this. Put your hands under hot water, and of course your hands will feel warmth. This is not the same as feeling the life-giving energy that can also produce a feeling of warmth. Energy the Chinese call Chi, the Japanese – Ki, the Romani – Di. Although this life energy can produce feelings of warmth, it is different from simply having warm hands.

I encourage you to experiment with feeling the energy around you. Feel the energy of different parts of your body, feel the energy of your family members, your pets, plants, and even furniture. Notice how different homes and outdoor environments have different energies. Have you ever toured a number of homes in a day and noticed how different the energy is in each one? This is a good way to test your ability to sense things. If you have a day of running errands, notice the energy of different neighborhoods, different stores, different people you encounter in a day. Everything has energy. Every place has energy. Every person has energy. Tune into it and soon you will be able to distinguish the negative and positive energy around you and choose more thoughtfully where you will spend your precious time.

Connecting to Health and The Kingdom

Shuvihano's energy exercises are all about energy exchange between you and the world. Let's say you'd like to get a pen to write a note.

Imagine you are sitting on a couch and the pen is on the table several feet from you. To get the pen, you have to get up, walk to the table, and pick it up. If you'd like to keep the pen, you'll put it in your pocket or hold it in your hand. If you don't like the pen or if it no longer works, you will throw it away.

The same principle applies to energy. If you'd like to get more energy, you have to get up, walk outside, stretch your arms, "pick up" the energy (the fact that you can't see it doesn't mean that it's not there), and either put it in your "energy pocket" (the area below your belly button) or hold it in your hands. Your energy needs to be connected to the energy of the Earth for you to experience complete health.

I know many different methods of "grabbing" good energy and keeping it (finding more and more different pens). You can grab the energy of the ocean, you can grab the energy of the Sky and the Earth. Many men benefit from grabbing the energy of the Sun, and women thrive when they are open and grab the energy of the Moon. The polarity is nice too – for women to know they are consciously pulling in the masculine energy and protection of the Sun, and for men to surrender to the magic of the feminine Moon.

And then there is the magic of making peace with the world of plants. I had a client who had become accustomed to carrying tissues around with her everywhere, in her briefcase, in her purses, in her car, by her bed, at her desk, because she constantly had colds and hay fever and experienced sensitivity to everything. She thought it was normal to need tissues everywhere and didn't even question this habit. She thought it was normal to have a shelf in the bathroom stocked with cold medicines and allergy drugs. After working with me, she came to understand that her diet, sleep, and the energy of her surroundings all needed to change. And the most important thing was for her body to be retrained not to react to the Plant Kingdom.

We worked together on this. The key thing that had been missing from her body needed to be addressed. She had to get energy from nature and be grounded in it. This may sound to you as if these illnesses and complaints are not connected, but they are—her body was constantly reacting to pollen and to bacteria and viruses constantly because she was indoors all the time, not part of the natural world, and her body was signaling her distress. Her soul was asking for more of being outside and more of being with the right people in the right places.

Some people in the same circumstance do the opposite thing their body is requesting—they spend even less time outside because they have allergies! But as soon as she walked outside barefoot regularly, ate many plants, drank beautiful fresh green juice, spent time hiking, got in the water of the ocean and lakes, and opened the windows to sleep with fresh air coming into her bedroom, all of her symptoms and illnesses went away. When you connect to the energies of the Kingdom and all of its energies – plants, stones, living water, wind, and all living things – your body and soul will rise in vibration.

Swimming in The Magic

Animals and fish are important parts of this energy that surrounds us. Different animals have different energies associated with them. Once I was offered the opportunity to swim alone with one of the most connected mammals we have to our consciousness–a dolphin. The dolphin had been named Lana, which was a very lucky "coincidence" for me since my name is Mi-lana. The energy exchange between us was so amazing I struggle now to find words to describe it. We talked, we played, we healed each other. I gave Lana a massage and she shared her healing sounds with me. Our exchange of energy put me in a different world. What happened there was beyond anything I've ever experienced.

The woman who took care of the dolphins said that during the winter when no one swims with the dolphins, they started to obviously miss being with people. They get very lonely and can even get sick from missing people.

During the summer, they spend the whole day swimming with people, healing them, helping them, playing with them, taking away their pain and negative emotions. Then winter comes and they feel the emptiness; they no longer feel useful or appreciated. This is a beautiful truth that plays out with other animals, environments, plants, and rocks too. We are in a dialogue with nature that we often just don't know about. Until we do. And now…you do!

Everything around us is alive. The wind greets us when we go outside, and it is delighted when we notice it and comment upon it. The wind throws our hair in our face to say, "Hello!" When the wind plays with my skirt, I play back by turning quickly to say thank you. The trees, bushes, fruit, vegetables, grasses are all waiting for our touch. A big beautiful green beetle flew around me as I ate lunch and I put out my arm calling for it to land and inviting it to say hello. Of course it did. Walked up my arm. I blew it a kiss and sent it on its way.

The natural world is as starving for an opportunity to teach us as we are for the wisdom of nature. The rocks do their best to support us, to give us strength and courage. They all have spirit and they are more than happy to help those who notice, who are aware, who are "in the know." That's how these conversations get started and how talismans are made. I ask an object to help me, to go to the spirit world on my behalf and create a desirable outcome. Eagles are the highest-flying creatures among us. When you see one, invite it to carry your prayers up and up. Everything around us is happy to help us. Let us be respectful and kind in return.

Love on Fire

For hundreds of years, Romanies have been getting energy from Fire without even realizing it. When you sit around a campfire, it is a natural reaction to stretch your hands closer to the fire. We take this a step farther and imagine the fire's energy entering through our palms and spreading all around our body. Grab a branch, hold it in the smoke, and then ask your friends or family members to brush it from your neck and down the spine. You will get a feeling as if butterflies are gently touching you with their wings. You are being kissed by the smoke, swept clean, and it will bless you.

Have some fun feeling your way around energy and play games with it. Where do you feel best? Where are the spikes of energy? Where do you find your feet picking up and your heart lifting? Notice where you feel good and spend time there and thank that place for being a place of peace and delight for you.

Pick and choose and experiment – the Universe has created all kinds of energy just for you. All you have to do is walk outside and grab it.

The same principle applies when you would like to release your negative energy. But instead of "grabbing," you will be "throwing away." In the beginning, I felt uncomfortable releasing my negative energy into the Earth. I didn't want the Earth to get all my energetic "trash." But soon I realized that the Earth gladly recycles it. It is not hurt by our release of negative energies. It is only hurt by the impact of our negative thinking and the actions we take when we are influenced by poor or negative energy. Once released, the negative energy can be recycled and upgraded through the natural processes of the Earth. If kept by us, it causes us much damage, not only to ourselves, but also to the world around us. But when we release negative energy into the Earth, it is transformed.

Problem: You are exhausted but have to keep going and need a quick pick me up.

Solution: Stand up straight and raise your hands above your head. Bend down and relax your arms, neck, and face completely. Close your eyes. You can bend your knees a little. Relax your cheeks, tongue, and eyes. Be like a cooked noodle, move your arms and head a bit, so that everything is loose. Stay here as long as you can without straining yourself. Come up. Stretch up as if you are trying to touch the ceiling. Rub your hands together as if you are trying to start a fire. Put your hands under very cold running water, splash some on your face. Drink a glass of live water. Take a deep breath and smile.

Mind Traveling Journey

Once, a taboro was looking for a village where families could spend the winter. When the houses of the first village became visible, the Rom in the first wagon saw an old man walking towards them. The Rom stopped the wagon and greeted the man. "Say, good fellow, what kind of people live in that village? We are looking for a place where we can spend the winter." The man asked in return, "What kind of people lived in the village where you spent last winter?"

"Good-hearted, generous people. We were sad to leave that wonderful village."

"This is the kind of people that live in this village," responded the man and kept walking.

I close my eyes in a dark, quiet room. I see a long corridor with a door that looks like an arch at the end. I am wearing Gypsy clothes. I open the door and enter a beautiful garden. I close the door behind me and memorize its location in the garden. It's located at the bottom of a small mountain; it will be easy to find. Suddenly, my clothes turn a bright white. I leave the beautiful garden and walk around in a meadow. I notice that there are lots of white daisies with yellow centers for as far as I can see. The Russian word for daisies is "romashka." Suddenly, I begin to think that the root of the word "romashka" is "roma." Roma – this is how Russian Romanies call themselves. But this is just my interpretation.

I walk for some time and then see an old man coming towards me. He has a gray beard and gray hair. I greet him warmly and we continue to walk together.

"Ask me anything you wish to know," he says.

I think for a few seconds and then ask him, "When someone is in pain, how can I take away that pain?"

He replies, "There are many ways. You can use a leaf of raw cabbage or a sliced raw potato. Place it on the painful spot. Wrap it and leave it there for a few hours. Or you can use your hands. Imagine that there is an eye on your palm. This is a very kind, loving eye that emit healing energy. Focus the healing energy onto the painful spot. If you need self-healing, stand in front of the mirror. Make sure you are in a good mood. If you are sad or angry, don't look into the mirror because it will cause a lot of damage. You see, eyes are the channels of energy. When you have angry eyes and look at other people, you send them negative energy. If they don't have a strong protective shield around them, they will get sick. If you have kind, loving eyes and look at other people, you will send them healing energy. When you look into the mirror, you can make yourself sick or healthy depending on how you gaze at yourself. Look at yourself with kind, radiant eyes and love what you see. Always smile when you look at yourself in the mirror. If you are sad, don't look in the mirror at all."

I am listening attentively and wonder if this is the reason that in Russia, when someone dies, all mirrors in the house are covered with fabric. I never thought about this before. All of this information is new to me, and I am trying to remember every word.

At this point, we come to a shore of a beautiful river. "This river has healing water," he says. "Take a plunge." I don't hesitate to jump into the river. It has a very strong current and I have to use all my strength to get back to the shore. I swim quite a distance, and when I come out of the water, the old man greets me again. *How could he have gotten here so fast?* I wonder. I am ready to continue the conversation, but I see a gorgeous horse running towards me. The horse is brown with a white stripe on its forehead. I can't keep myself from riding it. I jump on the horse and take off. The wind whistles in my ears and I have a feeling of absolute bliss. When I stop the horse I see the old man again. How did he get here so fast?

"It's time to go," he says. He leads me back to the beautiful garden. I open the door and go back through the corridor. I open my eyes. The mind-traveling journey is over, but the memory of it is as real as a memory of an actual life event.

I am looking at my birthmark that looks like a horseshoe. It's a sign of a Gypsy healer. When I looked up the meaning of the word "horseshoe" in the dictionary, here is what I found: "U-shaped protective metal plate fitted to the rim of a horse's hoof." "Protective" is the key word here. A horseshoe has been used for protection in Russian families for ages. It would be hung on top of the entrance to the house. To Gypsies, it has an even more sacred meaning. At first, I thought my birthmark looked like an arch. But now I see that it also looks like a horseshoe. So, when I go into my mind traveling journeys, I believe this mark on my body protects me. The door I use to travel between the worlds looks like an arch, and there is a horseshoe over it for protection. Go figure.

MIND TRAVELING JOURNEY RULES

For simplicity, I will call a mind traveling journey simply a journey. It is different from the mind traveling you learned earlier in this book. In mind traveling, you are making things up. You are in control. During journeys, you start by mind traveling, but then you begin "watching a movie" without knowing what will happen next. The journey is a real journey for your soul; even if you think you are making things up, and soon you will see that the Universe is showing you things. Start your journey by mind traveling to your favorite place in nature. Imagine a door that opens into this place. Remember where you started. You will have to go back the way you came in. You have to literally trace your steps back and find the door between the worlds. If you don't see the door, don't open your eyes. This is not a game. You don't want a part of your soul to become stuck there, in the parallel world.

You need to, you *must*, start the journey in a positive mood. If you are in a state of fear or sadness, don't do it at all. Your emotions during the journey will attract entities with similar emotions. Let me tell you, the entities in the parallel world can be extremely frightening. They will use every possible way to feed off your fear. And if you get scared and open your eyes, they will remain attached to a part of your soul. This is how phobias are born. This is why people are afraid of things that it is not logical to be afraid of, and to heal these fears we must use the opposite action that created that fear.

If you don't meet anyone during your journey (a person or an animal), try talking to the trees or any parts of nature that you see. If you don't hear a response to your questions, you are not ready to communicate with other worlds. Come back again later.

Please make sure you don't fall asleep during the journey. You stop being in control if you are asleep. It happened to me once, and it was the most unpleasant experience. I woke up from the strong shaking of my body. My soul was trying to leave my body and it created a state of shock. I also realized that I generated a lot of heat. Journeys in general generate a lot of energy.

Mind Doors

My daughter used to write stories about her cat Sapphira. In these stories, Sapphira travels the world, both the physical and the spiritual. Each sentence in the stories is loaded with hidden meanings. Here is one of her stories:

One day Sapphira got lost during one of her many adventures. She desperately needed help. She wanted to return home but did not know the way back. She was lost in the middle of a tropical island. Everyone she approached for help told her that only the King of the Island knew the way out, but alas, no one was allowed to speak with the King. Not able to speak with the King in person? Not a problem. She decided to enter his mind and ask for help this way.

First, Sapphira did a little dance. Have you ever seen a cat dance? She jumped up and down and ran around. Then she stretched out her paws, sat down, and closed her eyes. She began meditating, or as she called it, meowditating. Meowww, meowww… Some time passed and soon she saw a long corridor with several doors. She began reading the signs on the doors. After a while she saw a sign that read, "King of the Island," on one of the doors. Trembling with nervousness, she knocked on the door. Bing, bang, bong. Knock, knock, knock. The door slowly opened and she saw the King of the Island. "An unexpected visitor," said the King. "It's been a long time since someone visited my mind. You are a brave little kitty. What can I do for you?" Sapphira stopped trembling and asked, "Can you show me the way back to my home?" The King nodded his head. "Here is the map," he said, pulling out a piece of paper with a map of the island. "Here is the way to your house. Remember it well since the map only exists in your mind." Sapphira memorized the map, thanked the King, and went back to the corridor. She opened her eyes and smiled. She knew how to return home.

Problem: You don't see anything with your eyes closed.
Solution: It takes time to activate your inner eye. Close your eyes and *imagine* a circle. If you can't imagine a circle, imagine drawing the number one in the air. Try different shapes until you are certain you can see it. If you can imagine something, anything with your eyes closed, soon you will be able to see other things that come to you without first having to imagine them.

Places of Power

Once there was a peasant who was a good blacksmith and made amazing things out of metal, but he did not have many clients. He was poor and unhappy. One day he decided to leave his village in search for happiness. He searched in the valleys, he searched in the mountains, he searched in the seas, he searched in many different countries. In all his searching he wore out one hundred boots. He became old.

One day, as he was walking along a dirty road, he saw a blind beggar. He gave the beggar alms and sat down next to him to rest. The beggar asked the peasant where he had been and what he had seen. The peasant began telling him about each country he had visited, each place in nature he had walked through. The beggar sighed and said, "Oh, how unbelievably happy you are!" "Me, happy?" The peasant gasped. "Thank you, good fellow." "What for?" asked the beggar. "For teaching me a lesson." Elated, the peasant took off to return to his village.

Not all places in nature are created equal. There are some extraordinary places that hold great magic. Some places provide portals to universal knowledge, others have healing properties, and yet others display symbols that offer a glimpse into the deeper meaning of our existence.

AN ISLAND

It was my father's dream to visit Hawaii. Why this was so, I will never know, since he passed away before I heard his explanation. But somehow his passion for Hawaii transferred to me. Perhaps he whispered this love of Hawaii into my ear.

The first time I visited Hawaii, I immediately realized that this was one of the most energetically rich places I'd ever seen. Every cell in my body was full of energy and joy. I can best describe this feeling as being alert and aware. I felt as if I had just awakened after a long night of very a deep sleep, refreshed and energized. I had a feeling that something exciting was about to happen, and then it would. The Hawaiian Islands have many sacred places, and I have visited many of them. Some of these sacred places were only known to locals, and they were very surprised to see me there. It is easy for me to find a sacred place. I am simply magnetized towards it.

One time, I was climbing a sacred mountain on Maui. With each step my heart would beat faster and faster. I was so curious – what would I find on top of this mountain? Finally, I got to the top, but the trees were blocking the view. I took several more steps and … I saw deer. Many deer. I began counting and didn't finish. I'd never seen so many deer in my life. I walked towards them and looked into their eyes. I had a feeling that their eyes were intelligent. They were so beautiful and peaceful. Sacred deer on top of a sacred mountain–I was in heaven.

As I began visiting Hawaii every year in search of for Hawaiian ancient healing techniques, I began having visions and dreams about Hawaii. I had a vision of a true lomilomi practitioner teaching me. Once again, my intuitive skills (with the help of the Internet) led me to exactly where I needed to be at exactly the right time and with just the right person, Makana Risser Chai. Her grandmother was a Gypsy and she offered to help me. She gave me the contact information for a royal Kahuna, a Hawaiian shaman, who was a Master of lomilomi and a personal healer for the King of Hawaii.

I met the Kahuna during my next trip to Maui. He was so famous for his miraculous healings that I expected him to live in a mansion on the beach. But he lived in a tiny apartment, far from the beach. When I came in, he unfolded a massage table and placed it in the small kitchen/living room. I told the Kahuna that I was from Russia and he said he had previously treated two Russian scientists. One of them couldn't walk. He had lost all hope of ever walking again. When he arrived, he did not believe the Kahuna would help, since everyone else with multiple degrees after their names had failed. The man who wanted to be healed was simply curious as to what he would do.

The Kahuna had a reputation as a miraculous healer. After several hours of massage, the one who couldn't walk got up and began walking. He later told the Kahuna that he expected him to wave his hands in the air and say some magic words. He thought that's what shamans did. He was surprised to learn that the Kahuna was very well educated in the human anatomy and performed actual physical adjustments of internal organs and skilled manipulations of parts of the body. What the Kahuna did was as scientific as physics. Why didn't more people know about these healing techniques? Just like other energy work, it was *kapu* – a kept secret.

I learned lomilomi from the Kahuna. All indigenous traditions include the practice of massage. The Western society stresses the benefits of massage as a tool for physical relaxation and benefits such as improved circulation and flexibility, or as a tool for mental relaxation and stress relief. A key element in Western massage is the connection of physical touch to the physical body. But the most important aspect of the massage is a loving touch and the spiritual growth it supports. The intention of the person who gives the massage and the intention of the person who receives it create an energy match. Then, if both open up their hearts, the outcome of the session will be miraculous. The energy of love is recognized by the soul much faster than feeling the weight of the hands on the body.

Massage used to be, and I am sure will become again, an every day experience. I am referring to self-massage and massaging your family members, pets, and even plants! In our family, we give each other a massage every day. It is not a formal massage where you have to be on the bed face down (although sometimes we do that too). It is a massage of a body part that asks for it. Both the person who receives the massage and the person who does the massage benefit. We take turns. Hand massage has enormous physical and emotional benefits. When my mother came home from the cancer hospital, she was in a panic. She couldn't stop crying. My grandfather began gently massaging her hands. First, the middle of the palm using a circular motion. Then, the whole palm using the rubbing motion. Then, each finger using a pulling motion. Then – the wrist using a twisting motion. My mom stopped crying and became very calm. If one of your family members gets emotionally upset, try the massage and see the results for yourself. The physical benefits of hand massage come from the fact that different parts of the hand connect to different parts of the body. For example, while you can't massage your heart, you can massage the area on your hand that corresponds to the heart, and in response the heart will soften, relax, and become calm.

But massage is only one part of the healing tradition. Hawaiian lomilomi is connected to the physical exercises that build strength and endurance – the martial arts called Lua. The martial arts aspect is what I think caused these traditions to be kept secret. Access to this knowledge by someone with bad intentions could lead to a lot of destruction. On the other hand, knowing the secrets of lomilomi will do no harm. The most important part of this healing tradition – love – is simply absent from an evil heart, and the heart of a true healer is so pure that powerful miracles become possible.

Although secret knowledge has always existed and will always exist, I am forever grateful to the few who took the courage to share some of the secret healing techniques with the rest of the world. Whether or not we use them and how we use them will determine whether or not more secrets will be revealed.

IN ENGLAND

One day I was sitting in front of my computer when I heard a song in my head. The song – both the music and the lyrics – was very clear and precise. I felt as if the Universe was singing to me and I listened intently to catch it all. The song was so beautiful it seemed to arrive from a source far from this world. Like a sponge I absorbed every note and every word:

> The fairy tales of One Thousand and One Nights
> You'll visit the Castles
> You'll meet the Knight
> It starts today
> Go find the wheeler:
> Russian healer, Russian healer

Several words were repeated. They sounded like a mantra: "Russian healer, Russian healer." I experienced this as a special message for me, and so I immediately opened a search engine and typed "Russian healer." The first Web site that came up was about Alla Svirinskaya, a Russian healer practicing in London. I had already started writing my book about Gypsy energy secrets, so I was shocked to find out that she'd written a book with the same words in the title. Also, the name Alla has a special meaning to me. Alla was the healer in Alupka who taught me about living water. When I was a little girl, I had asked my mother why she didn't name me Alla when I was born. The name had significance to me, and I immediately felt the pull toward England.

I always follow the path of synchronicities with conviction because it is only through action that we get the life of our dreams. So I emailed Alla that moment and asked if I could come to London to meet her. Alla agreed right away. Everything fell into place over the next few days. I got my passport renewed in three days. I got a wonderful deal for the plane tickets and found an amazing hotel in London. I had a feeling that this trip would have a deep meaning in my life, so I searched for the most sacred sites in England with the help of the creative genius of my friend Lacy. I was ready to start one of the best adventures in my life.

ALL HALLOWS-BY-THE-TOWER

My first destination was one of the oldest sacred sites in London – the hill next to the famous Tower of London. This hill has been a place of worship for thousands of years. First the Druids, then the Romans came to worship here, and in 675 AD an Anglican church was built on the hill. This is now the oldest church in London. It was built on a place of very high spiritual energy. I have two energy rods that I took along for the trip. They show places of very positive, very negative, and neutral energy. When I used my energy rods inside this church, they registered very positive energy—off the charts energy.

I walked inside the church, looking at the statues and icons. When I reached the icons next to the altar, I saw unusual violet rays of light coming from above. They were not coming from the windows, and I wasn't able to pinpoint the source of these amazing rays of light. They felt like a shower of sparkling violet light penetrating one certain area in the front of the church. I couldn't get these rays on camera no matter how hard I tried. I stood breathless, enveloped by radiance, unable to move. I soaked up something very positive and very powerful. It was a gift of energy.

After several hours had passed, I reluctantly left the church and looked at the Tower of London. It was a place of torture, imprisonment, and execution. It was steeped in cruelty, sadness, and sorrow. Thousands of people stood in line to visit the Tower. I walked around the Tower with my energy rods and registered very negative energy. How interesting, all these people were spending their time and money to visit one of the most negative energy places in London, not knowing they would pick up those energies, while right next to it there was an empty old church, filled with highly energetic, positive, ancient goodness that could be pulled into the body and mind to enhance life. I look forward to returning to that church to pull in more light and love. And I encourage you to find it and other places like it on your journeys in this beautiful world.

ROLLRIGHT STONES

My next destination was the Rollright Stones. My wonderful friend Lacy warned me that it would be very difficult to get to the Stones without a car. First, I would have to take the tube to a train station, then take the train to Kingham, then take a bus to Chipping Norton, and finally I would have to walk for hours to get to the stones. Still, I was determined to get there. And so I set off on my adventure.

It was my first ride on an English train. The seats were very comfortable and it felt as if we were riding on the clouds, soft and smooth. I didn't know how much time it would take me to get to the town, so I looked around to ask someone for help. Behind me, I saw two old English gentlemen. They were drinking tea (I smiled) and discussing important matters with sophisticated English accents that charmed me. I asked them if they would let me know when my stop was coming up. They replied in the most polite way that certainly they would. They looked exactly like a modern Sherlock Holmes and Doctor Watson and this delighted me. I did not have any British reserve. I was smiling freely and not guarding my heart at all. What they thought of me was not my concern. I only sent them love. We parted as friends in my world.

I was the only one getting off at this place of Kingham. I took the bus to Chipping Norton. During the bus ride, I admired old houses and castles (were these the Castles from the song I heard before my trip to England?). At Chipping Norton I realized that I was supposed to cover a distance much longer than I had calculated at home. I had a map I had printed from the Internet, so I began walking. At some point I realized that I had lost my way. It turned out to be one of the most difficult walks in my life. The Universe was testing me, as it has many times before and would many times after this walk. But the journey was worth it. Journeys are always worth it.

I had done my studying before arriving. The Rollright Stones consist of the stone circle (The King's Men), a standing Stone (The King Stone), and a burial chamber (the Whispering Knights). The Knight – from that song I had heard again. The Rollright Circle consists of seventy-seven stones. Seven is considered a lucky number in Russian and Gypsy traditions. It is twice as lucky here. The stones are about five thousand years old. According to legend, they were once the army of a king who planned to conquer all of England. A witch turned the king, his knights, and his men into stones. Why? The legend is silent about that.

There are many legends tied to the Rollright Stones. Some say moving or chipping the stones will cause death (just like with dolmens), others say little folk (well-described in Gypsy fairy tale tradition) appear from underneath the stones at midnight.

I walked for many miles from the bus stop. Dark clouds gathered in the sky, a cold wind began to blow, and then it rained. I didn't have an umbrella or warm clothes. I kept walking without giving up. I raised my arm in hopes that the passing cars would give me a ride. Not one car stopped. Tired, cold, exhausted, and wet, I finally made it to the Stones. I walked inside the stone circle and oh, a miracle! The weather suddenly changed completely. The sun appeared out of nowhere, the wind calmed down, and the rain instantly stopped.

It was warm inside the circle. It was cold outside the circle. It was sunny inside the circle. It was cloudy outside the circle. It was dry inside the circle. It was rainy outside the circle. I used my energy rods and registered very positive energy inside the circle. I sat in the middle of the circle and felt absolutely blissful. I felt the union of the Earth, the Sky, and the entire Universe. I don't know how much time passed. I soaked in the positive energy and sent out my appreciation for this sacred place. Then, it was time for me to leave. I had to walk for several hours back to the bus station.

On the way back, I thought how wonderful it would be to rest and eat in some place warm. I walked for a few more minutes and out of nowhere appeared a sign "Tea House." The timing was magical. Did I become more powerful after visiting the Rocks? The Tea House was warm and served wonderful fresh food. I then resumed my journey back. I stopped next to one of the old houses that looked as if it was transported there straight from a fairy tale and admired its beauty. A window opened and a middle-aged woman with full pink cheeks appeared holding a hot pie in her hands. We smiled to each other and said hello. The woman asked me where I was headed. I told her I was going to the train station. She offered to give me a ride, she just had to turn the stove off. I protested – I didn't want the trip to be inconvenient for her. But she wouldn't take no for an answer. It was another miracle – I had missed my bus and would have had to walk for hours to the train station. It felt as if something changed after I visited the Stones. Happy "coincidences" became a norm. My heart was light and full and every conversation and encounter I had felt blessed.

MERLIN'S CAVES

My last destination was Merlin's Caves, commonly known as Chislehurst Caves. This site is thought to be more than 8000 years old. Caves are entrances into the Underworld. This is very serious. No joking about caves. Enter at your own risk.

I was told by a trained guide at the Caves that the Merlin Caves are haunted, and it certainly seemed so to me. There is a horse drawn on one of the walls by a man who stayed in the cave overnight. He slept next to a pool of water where a woman had drowned. He swore he saw the lady. To stop himself from losing his mind, he began drawing the horse. He kept drawing until people came to get him.

Recently two boys took the challenge to stay overnight in the Merlin Cave. They didn't make it through the night. At two in the morning, one of them began screaming. The second one had a seizure. They were both taken to the hospital. From that point on, it was illegal to stay overnight in the cave.

The energy in the cave is very heavy. It bends you towards the floor, it doesn't let you keep going. It sends you all kinds of challenges. No use to be brave and fearless. This energy is much stronger than all your courage. This was a cave with complicated energy, but I knew I could handle it so I went in for the adventure.

There are different kinds of caves. Some are places to go to recharge. Others seem to absorb negative emotions and feelings. If you are suffering from any negativity, consider going to a carefully chosen cave. Stop to feel the energy before you enter. Is it a good place for you to be? You will know. If you are meant to enter the cave, you will be able to leave all your negativity there. It will magnetize to the cave. You will come back to God's light clean and clear.

ALLA

I met Alla in her house in London. She turned out to be a very friendly, warm-natured Russian woman. I instantly liked her. She gave me the most wonderful treatment imaginable, but I am not allowed to tell you what it was. She made me promise that I'd keep it secret. Some secrets are meant to remain secrets after all. I am grateful to her.

*　　*　　*

It was time to leave England and come home. I didn't know that my adventures had just begun–and once adventures begin, there is no stopping them.

BRYCE CANYON NATIONAL PARK

I had promised myself that I would visit Bryce Canyon after seeing an unusual photograph. I kept my promise. I always keep my promises. Something wonderful happens when I do what I promise.

Bryce Canyon – the canyon of thousands of colors, the home to Magi, Sorcerers and Wizards. The positive healing energy of the place is literally off the charts. It is amazing. This place is unique, mystical, magical.

Local shamans guard the sacred underground water. It is not only alive, it also possesses magical properties. This water changes perception and consciousness. Unsuspecting visitors can only catch a glimpse of the ever-altering perception of the landscape by looking at the hoodoos (rock formations) during different times of the day. They change their color from grey to blue to pink to orange, and then to yellow, red, and purple. When the sun shines upon the rocks, they seem transparent. The canyon sings, and the song changes as the colors change. It sings of children of the Sun and the Wind. It sings of Gypsies.

As you walk along the canyons, not only do the colors and the sounds change, the pressure, the temperature, and the weather change too. I started one day at the top of the canyon. It was a cold, crisp morning. As I kept walking down, it started to rain heavily. I kept walking, wet to the bones. It suddenly became dry and very hot. Then windy and chilly. The canyon was playing with me, testing my determination and perseverance. It doesn't share its secrets freely. You have to earn its trust. Then you are initiated into the family of the Magi that know the secrets of altering time and space.

The Paiute Indians have a legend that Bryce Canyon used to be a city inhabited by Legend People. They were creatures who could make themselves look like animals or people. They were turned to stone by the powerful god Coyote as a punishment for making him angry. What did they do to make him angry? Just like in the Rollright Stones legend, this part of the story is not known. There are several versions, all very different from each other. But here it is again, a legend of people turned into stones, just like in Rollright Stones. Two very different nations. Two very similar stories. And one Gypsy woman on a quest to understand.

I sat down on a rock bench, closed my eyes, and listened intently. I tuned in to the whisper of the rocks, of the rock beings. They talked. They said, "People, do you know how happy you are? You can move! You can travel from place to place. This alone is enough for you to be happy beyond measure for the rest of your life. We are jealous of you, people. You are the lucky ones, although many of you don't understand this. Yet try it: stand next to us and keep standing as long as you can. Don't move, stand completely motionless, as if you are rooted to the ground. How long will you be able to stand like this? One day? What about one night? The wind will blow from all directions. The rain will pour from above. The heat will try to reduce you to ashes. Yet you stand, not moving. Yet you stand, completely motionless. Breathe in, breathe out."

The rocks also have a soul. The rocks also want to move. Those rocks that fall down the mountains – they are the lucky ones. They are able to move even if only for several minutes during all their long lives. In this they will gather many fleeting impressions to remember for the rest of their lives – for the next few million years. The rocks do not complain–no, they do not. They are surprised at how many of us don't understand happiness. The stones are alive and are able to read the thoughts of all people walking next to them. "Look, here comes a gloomy person. We are trying to cheer him up, to transfer our positive energy to him, but his head is so filled with his gloomy thoughts that he is not able to hear us. You can hear us because you are listening to us. A rare person is listening to us. Yet we are missing the communication with people. Come here often, listen to us, ask us about anything you wish. And tell us what you've seen that is beautiful in your life of movement. You don't even have to say a word. Simply imagine beautiful places in nature. The more beautiful your thoughts are, the happier we will become in our souls, the more joyful our rocky life will be. Come here often: we'll share our strong, powerful energy with you. We will share our secrets."

After this extraordinary communication with the rocks, I took a hike on one of Bryce's trails. I looked around, paying attention to the unusual shapes of the rocks. I saw people and animals; giants and dwarfs; praying nuns and queens; castles and houses; mushrooms and candles. Suddenly, I saw the rocks that looked like the Tower Bridge in London! I could not believe my eyes. It seemed that all my adventures were connected and were pieces of one puzzle that I was supposed to put together. I was in a playground and enjoying the way the Kingdom was playing with me. *How did those stones experience me and my energy?* I wondered. I walked barefoot to feel the soul of the place. I slowed down to have conversations with everything that was around me.

ZION NATIONAL PARK

I don't know why I dreamed about visiting Zion National Park. I always felt that this place was sacred. The Zion Canyon's Paiute name is Mukuntuweep, which means "sacred cliffs." But I didn't know that until I visited Zion. It will be the last adventure described in this book, and it was a monumental one.

The first day at Zion gave me clues that the discovery I was about to make there would be significant. The red rock cliffs were the biggest I'd seen in my life. I found out that the first known inhabitants of the land lived in the canyon over 8000 years ago, just like the Merlin's Caves dwellers. They were nomadic people gathering wild foods.

When I was a child, I played a paper and pencil game called Labyrinth. It involved two players. The first player would take a checkered piece of paper and secretly draw the labyrinth square using letters A through J and numbers 1 through 10. Inside the square, the first player would randomly place walls, holes, and one chest with treasure. He would then place the second player anywhere he wished inside his completed labyrinth. The second player would get a blank piece of checkered paper with a dot in the middle. The second player wouldn't know where in the labyrinth she was placed by the first player. The second player would then say out loud, "I'd like to go up." The first player, looking secretly at his drawing would say, "You can't, there is a wall," or "You fell into a hole." Then, after trial and error, the second player would hear the long awaited, "You found the treasure!" I felt like the second player in Zion. Someone placed me randomly in a natural labyrinth surrounded by monoliths. I was going up and down, bumping into walls and boulders, passing waterfalls and lakes, looking for that hidden treasure I came here to find and take home with me.

Just like in Bryce, I had to pass the test before the sacred knowledge would be shared with me. This test was climbing Angels Landing. This is one of the most strenuous hikes in Zion. The last part of the hike requires holding on to chains in order to not fall into the abyss. Once on top of Angels Landing, I felt as if I was on top of the world. The feeling that I was about to learn something life-altering was even stronger here.

Next, I hiked the Hidden Canyon. It involved holding on to the chains again, followed by bouldering. I enjoyed the Hidden Canyon so much that I wanted to find something similar, hidden from the visitors, involving a lot of bouldering. I searched around, away from the crowds. Finally, I found a deserted canyon along a dried out river. This was the most pleasant of all hikes in Zion. I didn't see a single person. It was completely deserted. I climbed several rocks, going farther and farther from the road. Suddenly, I saw something that made me freeze. I saw … a dolmen! A real, natural dolmen. I could not believe my eyes.

Dolmens are stone houses built three to ten thousand years ago. Dolmens indicate places of enormous power. A legend has it that dolmens were built by Giants for the Little People.

Think of a dolmen as an old phone booth. Do you remember old phone booths? You had to walk inside a phone booth, drop in some money, and then you could make a call. A perfectly working phone would be useless if you had no money. A dolmen is a connection to the universal information library. You can call and find out an answer to any of your questions; you can even connect to the most powerful healing energies.

Warning: these are places of extremely high energy. If I take my 110V blender to Europe and plug it in into their 220V outlet, it will burn up. Same is here: if your energy level is low, you may get very sick after visiting dolmens. You may even shake and cry while visiting dolmens. They will also reflect your emotional energies back to you. Destroying or chipping parts of the dolmens causes mysterious death. Visit dolmens with a pure heart and only the most positive intentions.

I took a deep breath and entered the dolmen with a feeling of exhilaration. I closed my eyes inside the dolmen and connected with the energy. "What is this?" I asked, "Why am I here?" I heard the response right away: "Many, many years ago, there were plenty of natural dolmens on Earth. They were created for people so that they could communicate with the Divine. They were open for all.

But certain people did not like that. They wanted to restrict the access to the Divine, to keep it to themselves, to gain the power so that the rest of the people would worship and fear them. They destroyed natural dolmens and built man-made dolmens. They controlled the access to the man-made dolmens by killing anyone who approached them it without permission. This is why there are so many human bones found next to the dolmens. These were not burial sites. These were the sites of access to Cosmic communication. The greatest gift you can give to people is to tell them to return to natural dolmens and to natural communication with the Divine. This means one-on-one communication. Return to everything natural: natural food created by nature and not altered by humans, natural water created by nature and not altered by humans, natural clothing, natural housing, natural gardening. This is the message we have for you."

I stayed there a bit longer, quietly contemplating what I had heard. I left the dolmen and walked back to the road. I felt that I had completed my mission and it was time for me to leave. This place was within relative driving distance from my home, and I knew I could come back here any time. To ask more questions. To learn more secrets. Roma say, "God ordered us to walk the world."

Problem: You think you don't have money to travel.
Solution: First, see if this is really true. Often people imagine that traveling costs more than it actually does. Do you waste money on experiences and things that aren't as valuable to you as travel would be? Are there opportunities to find new work or encourage good fortune that will support more travel? Actually take a moment to research the cost of going to places you have always dreamed to visit to see what it will take to get there. I know a young man with autism who travels the world alone, working odd jobs, making friends,

exploring with incredible courage, and if he can do it, you certainly can too.

If travel in the immediate future is not actually feasible, don't fret! You can still embark upon meaningful travels within your own proximate community. Explore your surroundings and see what other people come to your part of the world to see. Take a long walk beginning in your neighborhood. Go to the nearest park and search for edible weeds, flowers, wild fruit, and berries. Get your family or friends together and carpool to the nearest wilderness. Walk with awareness. Search for unusually shaped rocks. Touch trees, grass, notice small animals and bugs. Try to communicate with different parts of nature. What kind of thoughts appear in your mind? Can you feel your inspiration and creativity blossom?

The Gypsy Language is All in Puzzles; Learn the Language of the Universe

The first step in learning the language of the Universe is to accept that the Universe and all its parts have consciousness. Accept that there are no accidents. Notice "coincidences." Try to communicate with rocks, animals, and things in your house. Pay attention to your dreams. Heal your body, mind, and soul. This will increase the level of positive energy you have. The more positive energy you have, the easier it is to understand the Universe.

Because you will only receive messages and visions when you are tuned in to the Universe, you need to find your own way of tuning in. What works for me is simply trusting the Universe, being open to whatever is happening in the world around me, and choosing to be on the side of the creative forces of the Universe.

Actively search for messages from the Universe. Start every day with anticipation that you will receive a message from the Universe.

Start every day with awe and be open-minded. Search for beauty in architecture, music, art, and nature. Beauty is one of the ways the Universe gives us clues to powerful energy sources. Find your own way to move from mundane to sacred. Start searching for magic in your life and before long, magic will appear.

The better you know the language of the Universe, the better you will be able to interact with it. Learn the language of the Universe the same way you'd learn a foreign language. In the beginning, you will only understand a few words. Then, some phrases. Some time will pass and suddenly talking to animals, rocks, and inanimate objects will be as natural to you as talking to your friends.

But first you have to change your focus. We spend too much time in our heads and on our own concerns. We tend to drift off to the past or future, depending on our personalities. We think about hopes that did not come true, rehearse conversations with co-workers or friends, regret what we have done wrong, and imagine how we could fix everything. Most of the time as we are listening to someone, we have a simultaneous conversation in our head of *I would not do that in this situation, I hope he lets me talk now,* and so on. When you stop the constant chatter in your head, you notice the world as if seeing it for the very first time. You are paying attention to what's happening outside of you. You are genuinely interested in the people around you, nature, sounds, and surroundings. You don't focus on the thoughts in your head. Instead, you shift the focus to the outside world. You start noticing the most unusual things. And then the magic unfolds. Long ago, I noticed that trees have eyes, that many rocks are shaped like human heads, and that clouds are shaped like animals. Can you find this in nature too?

When you don't focus on yourself, you extend yourself beyond your body. The whole world with everything in it becomes a part of you. And then the Universe begins talking to you.

Once you learn the language of the Universe, your creativity will reach a new level. You will begin co-creating with the Universe, and every aspect of your life will be enhanced. You will begin using creativity as a tool for consciously manifesting your dreams. Romanies have always been very creative. Creativity is born from the union of imagination and passion.

If you feel stuck in your life and can't seem to move forward, start creating. Pick any form of creativity. At first you will be creating for yourself, not for others, so set aside any limits. Ask yourself, what would my soul like to create: a dance, a poem, a painting, a book, a garden? It doesn't matter what you pick and it doesn't matter how good you are. The most important part is the process of creation. Start actively creating instead of passively watching TV or shopping.

When you learn the language of the Universe, you will start to see the creation of the Universe in action, and you will start co-creating! Hidden talents will surface. You will somehow find time in the busiest of schedules to draw, or write, or dance, or sing… The Muse that governs the inspiration will be your best friend.

When you understand where you stand in the relationship with the Universe, you can start asking the Universe to make your wishes come true by using the language the Universe understands. When does the Universe understand you? When you feel the emotions of love, joy and gratitude. To make this process easier, I am offering you a special blend of essential oils found at the end of the book.

When you start appreciating what you have, the Universe begins to give you more. One time, my family was flying to Ukraine for a summer vacation. When we arrived at the airport, I kept thinking how much I appreciated the ability to fly anywhere in the world. My husband has a frequent flyer card that allows him to upgrade to business class if there is a seat available. I asked him to check if there was any availability. He refused; he didn't want one of us to spend the next ten hours without the rest. "Please ask them if they will upgrade all of us to business class," I urged him. My husband laughed. Our tickets cost $1,200 each. One business class ticket was $8,000. "Just ask," I begged. So my husband went to the counter and asked if there were any business class seats available. Yes, there were. Would it be possible to move all three of us? Yes, sure. I wasn't even surprised. I think a thought and it becomes true, so I have to be very careful about what kinds of thoughts I chose to think.

Imagine you think a thought and it immediately becomes true. For example, you think, "I am so fat," and there! You gain ten more pounds. Or you think, "The car behind me is too close, it's going to hit me," and there! It actually hits you. Track your thoughts for at least one hour (even better – for one day) with a notion of what would happen if EVERY single thought would become true. When my friend did this exercise, she was in shock! She was thinking too many negative thoughts! No wonder her wishes did not come true – the Universe was protecting her from herself! For the Universe to make your wish come true, you need to know how to translate your wish into the language that the Universe understands. Repeating a wish over and over will not make it come true. A wish will come true when it comes from your heart, not from your mind. It comes true when you are in the flow of love. Imagine it happening using as many details as you can while feeling love towards the entire Universe. Use the language of imagination and jump into the flow of creation!

Creative forces of the Universe use the same energy as the emotions of happiness and love. When you are in love with the whole world, all your wishes come true faster.

WISH ROOM EXERCISE

Pick your favorite room in the house and make it your wish room. When you have a wish that you would like to come true, go to this room, sit down comfortably, and surround yourself with the things you love most. Grab some pictures where you look young and happy, read some pages from your favorite book, remember something pleasant from your past. Do something, anything that will place you into the flow of love. And then imagine your dream coming true. Feel as if it has already happened. When your wish comes true, how would you look? What would you say? If you think you would jump or skip from joy, jump up and skip around the room. There are no rules when you are creating your own happiness.

While I don't have a wish room, I have a wish shelf on which I placed items that I love the most. I walk past this shelf every day and each time I pass it, I smile. You can create a wish night stand or a wish table. Put things there that you absolutely love, and don't forget to change them as you change.

Once you realize that wishes do come true, you will dare to dream big. You will be able to create your perfect life. What will you wish for? A perfect place for a home? A job you love? A soul-mate? I found the following saying in a fortune cookie (I love fortune cookies, they always seem to give me the message that I need during the specific time): "What the mind can conceive and believe, it can achieve."

CARPOOL

You can carpool with someone when this person's wish becomes your wish. Let's say your wishes come true very fast, but your husband's wishes don't. One day, your husband says he would like to go to Hawaii for free. Some time passes, but his wish does not come true. So your husband shows you some pictures of Hawaiian Islands, and you get excited about going to Hawaii. Now, you make a wish to go to Hawaii for free. Next week, your boss tells you that there is a conference in Honolulu that he would like you to attend. He will pay for the ticket, hotel, meals, and car rental. You check your frequent flyer miles and realize that you have enough miles for your husband's free ticket. You go to Hawaii together. For free. By the way, this is a true story: it happened to me.

All the techniques described in this book will dramatically increase your energy. Don't let it spin your head. You will suddenly feel very powerful. Use this power wisely.

A shepherd was sitting next to a small spring
  that was gently rolling its water down the hill.
  The shepherd was sad;
  his favorite sheep was taken by a river:
  it drowned in it.
  Having heard him complain, the spring says in turn,
  "Oh that river, that monster! It did it again?
  If I had so much water, I would not hurt a soul.
  I would flow down the valley, irrigating the meadow,
that's all."
  A week had passed and it began to rain.
  The spring turned into river, overflowing the terrain.
  It's bubbling, it's roaring, knocking down big oaks,
  flooding the village, drowning all.

Remember, it's easy to be humble when you don't have power. But when you have all the power in the world, it becomes very tempting to abuse it.

When you learn the language of the Universe, the mask you were wearing for a long time disappears. Wearing a mask takes a lot of our energy. Yes, being without a mask makes us vulnerable and can seem quite scary, but the benefits outweigh the risks. Opening your heart may seem like all of a sudden you have nerves on the surface of your skin. But removing the armor will make you so much lighter that you will feel like you are about to float! One of the things you will notice is that you will start to breathe more fully, as if the air became sweeter, as if you are standing next to a loaf of freshly baked bread. Your body language will certainly change. No more slouching, no more avoiding eye contact, no more looking down at the ground and crossing your arms around you. You will feel like your heart is ready to jump out of your chest! You have so much to give to other people! You are the one who will make the difference in the world. Suddenly, you will notice that people want to be around you. That they are drawn to you like the moths are drawn to a flame. You will become a storyteller. And your stories will bring smiles and laughter. Even the tone of your voice will change. It will become soft and sweet. You will talk slower and quieter, but more people will hear what you have to say. Little, mundane things will seem like a joy to do. You will notice so many details that you will be surprised over and over again: How come you have never noticed them before? You will stop to admire a beautiful flower, you will try to touch a rainbow, and you will enjoy listening to the rain.

And because you will be so in tune with the creative forces of the Universe, "coincidences" will begin to happen that will make your life seem magical. You will be "in the flow," or "in the zone." You will get your dream job. You will meet your soul-mate. You will start getting gifts for no reason. You will suddenly learn how to talk to the animals and even the trees. Your kids, pets, and plants will be the first to notice and appreciate the new you. You will have a sudden desire to skip once in a while. You will become spontaneous. You will have an abundance of new ideas. You will invent something. Your dreams will change. You will also start being kinder. You will start doing random acts of kindness without expecting anything in return. You will realize that you are able to heal and to comfort. To get someone out of depression. To save someone's life.

Some time will pass and you will constantly be in the flow of love. Everyone will notice that. The Universe will notice that and will make your wishes come true. You will become a different person. Your eyes will give you away. Your eyes are the mirror of your soul. The smile will start in your eyes. Your tone of voice will change. You will be talking in a way you'd read a fairy tale to a child. As a storyteller, I've mastered it well. The energy of the whole room changes as soon as you change your tone of voice. Your posture will also change. You will walk into any room and light it up. Your soul will bloom like a beautiful flower.

In Russia, the word for "soul" is the most important word to people. You will know that the person is falling apart when "the soul hurts." (In English, the Russian phrases that contain the word "soul" are translated with the word "heart." Russian "from all my soul" becomes "from the bottom of my heart." A "soulful person" becomes "warm-hearted person." "Soulful conversation" becomes "heart-to-heart talk").

The best weather is "soul-touching weather." There is also a Russian phrase "the light of the soul" used to describe a spiritual person. When you are in pain (physical or emotional), don't let it turn off the light of your soul. No matter what happens, don't let it crush your spirit. Your body can go through a lot of pain, yet your soul can be shining with bright light. Your soul cannot be damaged or destroyed. It cannot be harmed even by the most severe pain.

You will open your heart and find you soul's purpose. To me, finding my soul's purpose came from knowing the language of the Universe. Our souls do not live in our bodies. Their home is in the "body" of the Creator of the Universe. By learning the language of the Universe, you learn the language of your soul. You will learn that happiness is following your soul's purpose and creating the world around you with love and gratitude. Power is when you are in charge of living your passion and making dreams come true without hurting anyone or anything in the world. Wisdom is understanding the laws of the Universe and believing in their fairness.

Coincidence at Will

I like to have client sessions outside. It helps ground them and we always get great results. One day I walked with a client who could barely walk. He moved very slowly, stopping and coughing. He was recovering from pneumonia and other illnesses and had been very ill for many weeks. He'd been in the hospital, flat-lined several times, and had been in a coma. He said that he had seen his relatives who had passed away when he had been on the other side with them. They said he had to stop destroying himself. What was he doing to destroy himself? Drugs, mostly meth. I knew this would be a tough conversation because he had to face things that would be hard in order to change his life, so I created the most beautiful light around myself and encompassed the man inside this warm light. He smiled and looked up. He noticed the sky. He started asking me about my spirituality, my teachings. He literally began changing in front of my eyes as his face softened and his internal light increased. Sometimes the best healing comes from just shining your light so brightly that it becomes contagious. I asked if he was experiencing any "coincidences." He said all kinds of spiritual books were appearing around him but that he had such a hard time with his former church that he was ignoring them. He had received diagnosis after diagnosis, including diabetes, and still he would not stop. It took literally dying to get him to pay attention. I explained how important it was to listen to the messages he had received from his dead relatives and to pay very careful attention to the "coincidences" in his life, including reading all of the spiritual books that had been appearing in his world. He did as I requested. We cannot ask for help and then turn it away once it arrives, or else the Universe won't take our requests as seriously.

I know a woman who put her passport on her altar and prayed a mighty prayer every day, wishing that she could have more international adventures with her family to deepen the connection between her, her husband, and their two teenage sons, and to have more educational experiences to inspire them as a family. The next week, a friend invited her to be in Bali in December, and her answer? A quick and hard, "No!" because...and I am not kidding when I tell you this was her answer...she was committed to be with her husband and boys in the U.S. in December for the holidays. Until it was pointed out to her, she hadn't even realized that she could ask if her family could join her on the trip. Do you see? An opportunity was arriving like a gift wrapped in a big bow, but she missed it. This is how we run and hide from the magic that is trying to find us. We don't listen for how the Universe wants to answer our wishes and prayers, and so we don't recognize the richness of the possible gifts that show up.

During my journeys and the bodywork with the shaman healers, I always have visions of different animals. One shaman told me that any time I have a vision of an animal I can look up its meaning in the book *Animal Speak* by Ted Andrews. For example, seeing a dolphin is a message for me to become more playful. Later, this book became my dictionary for the language of the Universe that involves animals.

Once, I had a vision of a white horse. Soon, I would find a white horse everywhere. My screen saver at work would display a picture of a white horse running on the beach with a heading "The Mystical Journey." I would get a chance to go horse back riding and one of the horses would be white. I would see a white horse on TV, I would hear songs about horses, someone would give me a calendar with horses, I would see a white pony giving rides to children. And you know how important horses are to Gypsies. From *Animal Speak* I knew that it was a sign that more and more magic would appear in my life. I would enthusiastically share these "coincidences" with my friends. "Isn't it wonderful," I would say, "to see how the Universe is communicating with us?"

But my friends didn't share my excitement. I quickly realized that different people have different interactivity with the Universe. Some have high interactivity, some – low.

To measure the level of your interactivity with the Universe, think of an object (for example, a feather), a concept (for example, success), or a person you rarely see. Sit down, relax, take a few deep breaths and imagine what you picked as clearly as you can. Send the energy of love to this image. Feel the magic of the process, then open your eyes and write down what you picked along with the date. Notice when you first see the object you chose, read the word you selected or hear it in a conversation, see or get a call/e-mail from the person you picked. Write the date down. Repeat this process several times to get an average estimate of your interactivity. If it took several minutes for the object to materialize, you have a very high interactivity. Several days – medium interactivity. Several months – low.

Once I picked the word "homeostasis." I'd read it in a book, but didn't understand its meaning. Instead of looking it up in a dictionary,

I decided that I would let the meaning of this word come to me. The next day, I went to the library to pick a "cookbook" about preparing raw foods. There was only one book on living foods on the shelf. All others were checked out. I didn't know anything about the author, so I decided to read a few pages. And there it was, right on the second page, the word "homeostasis", along with its definition! Did I mention it was a cookbook? But there were even more "coincidences" related to this book. When I had a vacation on Maui, I met a wonderful healer. She ate only raw food for fifteen years, so I e-mailed her about the book I found in the library. Turned out, the author was her neighbor and a friend!

Then one night, I had a vision: I saw myself in a beautiful white skirt and a white blouse. The next day, I received a magazine with an outfit just like the one I saw in my vision, right on the cover page!

Another night, I received an e-mail from my friend Olga saying that she had moved to Holland. I came home and learned from my husband that he had planned a business trip to Holland and would like me to go with him!

I will also never forget the lunch on a Sunday afternoon at an Italian restaurant. My husband and I were speaking Russian as usual. We had just come back from a hike in the mountains where I always get my inspiration. We talked about this and that and then I said, "I want to go to the opera; I REALLY want to go to opera." I just said it as a wish. Maybe, someday, sometime in the future, we would go to opera. I smiled, picturing this day in my mind.

Here is what happened next. A waiter came over to the table on my right. Suddenly, he started singing! He was singing an aria in Italian from an opera. He was clearly a professional singer. His voice was incredibly strong and beautiful. I didn't have to go to opera – the opera came to me.

When the number of "coincidences" increases, you'll know that you are moving in the right direction to the land where wishes come true. What if there are no "coincidences" in your life? It means that you are not moving at all. You simply don't know where to go. You are not following your soul's purpose.

You'll know you are on the right track in your life when you stop getting sick and experiencing pain and the number of "coincidences" increases. Any positive pattern is approval from the Universe. Life suddenly seems very easy for you. You find things that were lost a long time ago, you seem to avoid traffic or find parking spaces easily, you get a raise, and so on.

It is very important to notice "coincidences." When a "coincidence" happens, pay attention to it. Did you think of a friend you rarely see and suddenly you meet her at a grocery store? Were you thinking about buying a book and find it in your mailbox in a few days? Or maybe you remembered a certain movie, then turned on your TV at night and saw this movie? Remember these "coincidences," talk about them, write them down. Act on them by listening for what they are telling you. The more we listen and answer, the more magic shows up. Imagine them happening more and more often, and before you know it, they will.

Some of the "coincidences" will be just for fun; others will help you solve a problem. Below is one of the most unusual "coincidences" that I had.

One night, I saw myself dancing in a flame. The flame was inside a circle. I was not hurt by the flame at all; I even enjoyed this dance. As a Gypsy, I am used to dancing around the fire but never IN the flame. The vision left me puzzled. I wanted to find out what it meant. In the morning, I logged into the web site "Spirit of Ma'at" and noticed a new edition of the magazine about Russia. I was interested right away in the story written by Carol. I wanted to read more about her and jumped to her web site. I looked at her paintings and immediately noticed one with people dancing in the flame inside a circle!

I e-mailed Carol and asked her to explain this painting to me. She wrote back. It turned out the painting I saw was a vision for her as well! She wrote that seeing yourself unconsumed by flame represents life force or life potential, and the circle represents the Whole or Unity. No doubt I was feeling unity with the whole Universe!

Problem: You are following your passion but don't notice any coincidences.

Solution: They do happen, they always do, but you just don't notice them because your mind is constantly occupied with chatter. Focus on the outside world instead of on your own thoughts. To do that, change the way you do routine, mundane things. If you do everything the way you've always done it, you turn on the autopilot and your attention goes inward. If you start doing things in a completely new way, your attention goes outward and you start noticing things you ignored before. Stand on one foot when you are doing your dishes; take a different route to work; drive to an unfamiliar neighborhood and take a walk; go to the library and pick up a random book; start a conversation with a complete stranger; clean a drawer you haven't opened in ages; call an old friend; join a new club; go to a free lecture. If you are truly following your soul's purpose, you will start noticing "coincidences" left and right.

*   *   *

A soul's purpose is not something you can create now. It is not something you decide "fits you" or "makes sense." It is not something YOU make up.

Before you were born, you made an agreement with the Creative Forces of the Universe that you will follow a certain life path. You may then choose from many different ways to walk your life path, but you are not allowed to break the agreement and choose a different life's purpose.

Your heart knows it. Your subconscious knows it. But most importantly, the Universe knows it. Maybe you just never took the time to think about your soul's purpose. Or maybe you know your soul's purpose but think that if you follow it you will not be able to pay the bills. Maybe you were suppressing it for such a long time that it seems you forgot it. Ask yourself: What is it that I really, REALLY like to do? What do I do with ease and with love? What makes my heart jump out of my chest? What gives me butterflies in my stomach? If I could wish for anything, what would I wish for? If I had all the money in the world, how would I spend my free time? (Well, after you bought your dream car and a house on the beach of course).

(As a side note, if you answered, "I would just watch TV all day," this book is not for you. This book is for active co-creators of the Universe).

Remember the secret I told you earlier in the book? Were you paying attention? It is important, it is EXTREMELY important to make your childhood dreams come true. All children remember the agreement they made with the Universe before they came here. If you didn't make your childhood dream come true, you are blocking yourself from the opportunity of a life time.

Were you dreaming of becoming a singer? A ballerina? A ranger? You had your childhood dream for a reason. It doesn't matter if you weigh two hundred pounds more now. Sign up for that adult dancing class. Start singing in the shower. Take horse riding lessons. Something absolutely wonderful happens when you make your childhood dream come true. It is as if you have a magic wand but it is not working. After you make your childhood dream come true, all you have to do is wave the magic wand with your hands and miracles begin to happen.

My friend once asked: "What if my dream was to study leopards in Africa?" Here is what I said, "Today, buy the most beautiful picture of a leopard you can find. Hang it on your wall. Buy a stuffed leopard and put it on your bed. Go to the library and find all the books they have on leopards in Africa. Take small steps to bring your dream closer to you. Tell everyone how much you are fascinated with African leopards. The next thing you know, you will get a phone call with an invitation for a two-week safari trip. If you announce to the Universe your dream, the Universe will arrange for it to come true."

In two days, just to support my point, I got a postcard with a picture of a cat (my friend's nickname), a picture of a computer with the word "Internet" on it, and a picture of a leopard. I called my friend right away. "I have a message for you," I said, "Open a search engine on the Internet and type in 'leopards in Africa.' This is your first step. If you make it, the Universe will let you know the next steps that will help you to make your dream come true."

Remember, until you find your soul's purpose, you will feel restless. You will often feel an urge to go somewhere or do something. You will not know where to go or what to do, yet this urge will keep growing into a burning desire to change something in your life. Don't numb this desire with food, alcohol, or drugs. Don't turn it off by turning on the TV. It's a sign that your soul is desperately trying to get your attention. It is time to tell the truth to yourself. Who are you? What did you come here to do?

This book is about love towards the whole Universe and everything in it. And if it makes your inner light shine brighter, I have done a good job. I don't have enough words to express everything I'd like to say. It would be much easier to gather a group of people around me in a circle and start storytelling. The tone of my voice and the fire in my eyes would express so much more! But this book can reach many more people - that's why I decided to write it.

It is raining right now and every rain drop reminds me of perfection. Every drop is perfect in its shape and its purpose. You are just as perfect. Rain inspires me to write, just as you, my readers, inspire me to keep writing.

I am writing this book for everyone who is able to feel love. When I am writing, I feel a little sun lighting inside that keeps getting bigger and bigger, and suddenly I am the Sun. It is such a happy feeling – to shine and to give light to other people.

Before, when reading books, I did not understand: Why use so many words to express one idea? I understand it now: Words create an energetic chain that connects the writer and the reader. While you are reading this book, we are together, even if you are thousands of miles from me. Every new word allows me to deepen the connection. Words are energy. I have transferred my positive energy into the words of this book.

I was writing this book with so much love in my heart! This book is a gift to you, my dear reader. I've been noticing lately that I bring good luck. I have such a strong healing energy that it affects everyone around me. Because I poured so much of my love and energy into this book, this book will also bring you good luck. Think of this book as a Gypsy talisman I have created just for you.

Right now, this very second, beautiful music is playing. When I hear music, I start imagining things. Do you? I see myself riding a horse, collecting wild flowers in an endless meadow, dancing a Gypsy dance... Suddenly, my daughter walks into the room and starts reading a poem she just wrote:

A Gypsy Tale

Once coming from a foreign land
Telling future from a hand
Living in such sacred ways
Getting help from sunny rays.
Fancy dresses, long and wide
Money hanging from each side
With a horse coming so far
And the eyes each like a star.
Nature is their old best friend
Luck is what they wish to send
Not afraid of dark and night
In the forest they can hide.
They have powers, some of the best
They know that, no need to test
Gypsies have their way of life
Filling hearts with warmth and love.

The End, Or The Beginning?

There are books we hold in our hands that speak to us and give us just what we need, once, twice, or many times. Others pass through our hands like living water—we read and skim and drink deeply and then they are gone. A book can be something we read for information and then never touch again or a dear friend we share with many others.

I give you this book to be whatever you need and want it to be. It can be a game to play, a song to sing. I see a vision that some will gather in groups to read it together. I see how the ways of being that are shared in this book will benefit families and friends. Gypsies don't put things on the floor, so it will please me if you remember that this book should live on a beautiful table or be tucked onto a favorite shelf.

Whenever I think of this book and the ones who read it, I will send you my loving energy so that my desire to be of service to you is transferred through the words. There are no real endings or beginnings, just things flowing into each other.

A New Beginning, Again

I hiked in the forest expressing my joy and my gratitude for the abundant life force around me, below me, and above me in a place full of magic. I had just come through another difficult time and had emerged in my full Gypsy voice and with complete well-being— again. I had regenerated myself and I was celebrating!

Somehow, because I am as human as every other human, I had neglected to practice what I knew of Gypsy wisdom—again. I had slipped and fallen into an ordinary life—again! My real clothes in beautiful colors and textures were in the back of the closet, the most beautiful and precious things in my kitchen had been packed away and hidden. I had withdrawn myself from the world. I was wearing gray and living a gray sort of life. Even me. It was predictable that this would lead to a drop in my energy and health. It did. Even with all I know about how to live well, I had slipped in my practices and had become *regular* rather than *magical*. I had become overwhelmed and alone and full of self-judgment. I had not reached out to my taboro and was suffering alone. I was neglecting the Romani way of caring for myself. I wasn't attending to my surroundings in order to provide the environment of magic for the people I loved. *I teach this, I should know better!* I thought with self-judgment. But through this time of letting go I had also experienced a new level of compassion for my clients.

It takes time to develop a new positive way of being, and sometimes we test our own commitment by letting things slip so we can learn again what we are most committed to creating. I had gone through a time of experiencing disappointment, anger, judgment, depression, and loneliness.

The months before, I had been living at such a high level of energy and joy that it was a good reminder to slip down and hit the bottom again and to choose to dance my way into the light. We can learn to catch ourselves. When I felt the impact of where I was, I did what I recommend to my clients. I recommitted to do better and began again with self-forgiveness and a sense of humor. I laughed at myself and the predicament I had created. I would reclaim the magic by looking into my eyes in the mirror surrounded by candles. "I love you. Hold your head up and stamp your foot. Turn up the music. Sparkle. Shine. Demand. Hope. Wish. Wish. Wish!" I told myself.

Every new dawn is a chance to begin again. Expect magic, and miracles will fall out of your dreams and onto your pillow in the morning. Enjoy the dance of getting things in your life in order again. Love yourself in the midst of having life fall out of order, and then get it back in order and celebrate the recreation of you. I am both a teacher and a student, and I invite you to claim that for yourself as well. Sit in both roles. Learn and teach. Grow and share.

On this beautiful and bright day in the forest, I celebrated that my life was back in order! I was living in full color again! I recommitted to being fully myself and to doing my work with my whole heart. "Take your own advice," I sang under my breath with a smile. I could have sworn I heard a tree answer, "Yes, please do."

I will practice the old ways—again and again. I will continually restore my joy and health. I will let myself connect deeply with trees, flowers, animals, birds, insects, and the beating heart of the forest. I will take deep breaths of the fresh air that fills my lungs and drink the living water that is full of the energy of everything in the Kingdom.

I danced and turned around a tree, holding onto a branch as if it was my dance partner. I sat on a big stone that held me like a loving parent. The trees were dripping with berries. They were waiting for me to pick them. Dark blue berries and bright orange ones. Very sweet for my pleasure and very bitter for my health. I mixed them in my bucket and ate them together. That's how life is, always bitter-sweet. Trees thrive without interference and without regular water. I can learn even from this. The nutrient-rich, wild and free berries filled my belly and the basket I held in my hands as I skipped on the road, aware that if anyone drove here they could see me. I thought of my family, my taboro, my clients, my readers–how much I love them all, and you, and how much I want each of you to know the magic of life. "I will create right now that someone is delighted by seeing my own delight and stops to talk to me." Almost an instant later a car with a family pulled over to wave and have a conversation. They wanted to know what I was doing running around with my hair blowing in the wind, my bare feet happy in the grass in the mountains. "Foraging, and playing with the Kingdom!"

I doubt the family will forget their encounter with the joyous wild woman in the woods who was eating what she found with the joy of a daughter reconnecting with her beloved parents of Earth and Sky. We had fun together as the only humans in the woods. They clearly loved what they saw in me. And I loved them in the way total strangers can sometimes touch your heart so deeply. You see, we choose what we initiate and recreate and invent every morning. We get to invite the kinds of people we want to love, play, and work with into our magical realm. Everyone can, no matter the situation, circumstance, health, or wealth they experience, be in a creative dance with the Universe. Where you start doesn't matter. How many times you fall doesn't matter. Forget what came before and live as you wish–now.

You have the information on these pages and you have the practices and inspiration. I've shared stories to show you what's possible. You've seen that there are simple actions to take that will change your life for the better in an instant, and you have practiced them so that you know they are effective. You can always return to the study of what serves your life and continue to grow and reach up higher and higher.

When you sing, sing for the Kingdom. When you cry, give your heart fully. When you cook, add appreciation to the dish. When you love, let love also come to you from people, animals, trees, and rocks. God gave Roma the destiny of "roads and fair wind to our backs, water for fish, sky for birds, and the wandering path."

You are a powerful part of creation, and so naturally you too know how to create. The Universe is waiting for you. Your life is your own to make of it what you wish.

Join me on this ongoing journey of creating a passionate, healthy, and full life with Gypsy magic. I am here for you. I am always here for you.

Let's dance!

Eleven (Optional)

HEALING OILS

This section of the book is optional. The essential oils that I recommend are expensive. If you can't afford them now, don't be upset. I used to be so poor that I could not afford more than one meal a day. If you complete all the exercises in this book, life will change for the better. Suddenly money will find its way to your hands, and then if you so desire, you will be able to afford these essential oils as a complimentary means to increasing your abundance even more. You can also ask your family and friends to give you these oils as a gift, or you can get a group order and share.

*   *   *

Essential oils are the result of concentrating the purest essence of a plant into something that can be more powerful than using hundreds of that same plant. The powerful essence of essential oils lies in the fact that only the most magical and energetic part of the living plant is manifested into the oil. Simply put, a bottle of essential oil is pure goodness. What can be achieved through hours of meditation can also be achieved in a shorter amount of time through the use of essential oils. Essential oils have been used for thousands of years in healing, meditation, and other energy practices. Given their pure nature, they used to be extremely expensive and highly valued, used only by the royal families who could afford them. Now they have become more and more accessible, allowing anyone to expedite their connection to the Universe.

That is not to say that you can start using essential oils, instantly connect to the Universe, and that will be the solution to all your problems. Your connection and communication with the Universe is still reliant upon positive thoughts, listening to the world around you, and all the other techniques described throughout this book. However, once that connection is created, it can be further strengthened through various other means, including essential oils. Essential oils are not the be-all, end-all way to achieve a superordinate connection with the Universe. If you don't think that essential oils are for you, don't worry! You can easily find other ways to further connect to the Universe and manifest your energies. Keep practicing the techniques in this book, and your quality of life will improve significantly.

Now if you're like me, essential oils may just be the perfect addition to your routine. Not only are they extremely powerful and useful, but they can also allow you to maintain positive energy and a connection to the Universe when you may not have the time or energy to do so otherwise. As hard as I try to wish away an excruciating headache, sometimes I just can't gather enough strength to do so. Rather than continue suffering (or turn to harmful, artificial drugs), I can use essential oils to take care of the headache and then continue my day, spreading love and following my soul's journey. Some days I don't have the time to sit outside for a long time connecting to nature, so instead I use my essential oils. Think of them as a shortcut when you can't always afford going down the long path in your life.

* * *

Remember I said that not all places in nature are created equal? Not all essential oils are created equal either. There are some extraordinary essential oils that hold great magic. I've been using essential oils for many, many years, and through trial and error I have found what I believe to be the best ones and what I will recommend to you. If you'd like to see what I use every day, go to https://www.youngliving.com/, pick your country, click Become a Member, click "I was referred by a Young Living member, and I have his or her member number," enter Sponsor ID and Enroller ID as 1449556, complete membership info, and select Starter Kit (the best one is the premium kit with 10 oils and a dewdrop diffuser). After you receive your starter kit, you'll be able to choose any other essential oils and receive 24% off. Contact me at Gypsysoul2014@outlook.com if you need help.

Essential oils provide a shortcut to magic. They change your state of mind within seconds. If you've never used essential oils before, I recommend three books: *Essential Oils Pocket Reference*, Fifth Edition is the best place to start. *Ultimate Balance* by LeAnne Deardeuff is excellent too. *Essential Oils Desk Reference*, Special Third Edition is for advanced readers.

Unfortunately, the dark spirits are very real and very powerful. I will not be surprised if this book is banned at some point and the oils go out of stock. Get them while you can. Use the Angelica oil to protect yourself from the evil eye. Use Sage to cleanse yourself from curses.

The easiest way to use essential oils is to put a few drops on your hands, rub them together, and cup your nose. Breathe in, then open your hands to breathe out. Repeat several times. Read the labels to learn which oils must be diluted and which ones can be taken internally. You can also use a special diffuser sold with the oils to create a magical atmosphere in your home.

Essential oils that come from trees possess extraordinary ability to awaken psychic powers. Frankincense is the king of oils. Put a drop on your third eye to awaken your inner vision. Put a drop on top of your head to connect with your Higher Self. Use Sacred Frankincense for your meditation/prayer/shamanic journeys. Use Cedarwood for deep relaxation. Educate yourself on the use of Copaiba, Blue Cypress, Sandalwood and Balsam Fir. There is deep power in these oils that you will have to discover for yourself.

High quality essential oils added to a meal will turn it into medicine healing your body. Here are the ones I recommend: Rosemary to stay focused, Peppermint to stay alert, Oregano during cold season; Clove, Ginger, and Nutmeg to spice up your life. These are very concentrated oils. One drop goes a long way. Use DiGize with every meal to support healthy digestion. Just rub a few drops all over your stomach.

Don't add essential oils sold in regular stores to your water. It is not safe. The easiest way to add life to water is to add Vitality essential oils to it. Here are the ones I recommend: Lemon Vitality, Grapefruit Vitality, Ginger Vitality, Lemongrass Vitality, and Peppermint Vitality. Just one drop per glass of water. Stir fast. Never add essential oils to water in plastic containers.

It took me several years to buy all the oils I am recommending for you. I order one bottle each month. When they come in a package, I open them as if I am opening a Christmas present. I have hundreds of them now, my little helpers and Guardian Angels. Don't let the information below overwhelm you. One bottle of essential oils is better than nothing. It will last you a whole year. Pick what you need the most. Create a magical community and share.

To support feminine energy, use Clary Sage or Lady Sclareol during the first part of your moon and Progessence Plus during the second half. Masculine energy is supported by Mister and Spruce.

When I want to support my brain, I put several drops of Brain Power and rub them on my temples and the back of my neck.

When I want to support my heart, I put several drops of Aroma Life over the heart area.

When I want to support my muscles, I rub them with Elemi, Cool Azul, and Aroma Siez.

When I want to support my thyroid and adrenals, I put several drops of EndoFlex on my right hand and rub my neck, then I add some more and rub across the middle of my back.

When I want to support my liver, I rotate JuveCleanse and JuvaFlex. I put several drops on my right hand and rub my stomach on the right side under the rib cage.

When I want to support my kidneys, I put several drops of Juniper on my right hand and rub my back on the left side, then put several drops on my left hand and rub my back on the right side.

When I want deep peaceful sleep, I put several drops of Peace & Calming II, Lavender, or Marjoram on the soles of my feet, my temples, the back of my neck and my wrists. If I want memorable dreams, I use Dream Catcher in the same way.

To support my inner child and create the atmosphere of serenity, I use Gentle Baby. I put a drop on my pillow, on a cotton ball, on my face, and on my neck.

When work gets tough and overwhelming, I use Stress Away to calm down and Bergamot to regain my happiness.

When I want to stay healthy during the cold season, I rub ImmuPower on the soles of my feet.

To eliminate offensive smells and clean the air, I use Purification.

When I need an extra boost of energy, I use En-R-Gee.

Since I chose to live a long and healthy life, I rub Longevity just below my knees, on the outside of my legs.

I would also like to offer you several spells for use with essential oils. These spells were created to be used with the essential oils you purchase following the above instructions using the number 1449556. It adds up to number 7 and is blessed to support the spells. These spells should be used only with the most positive and healing intentions and are meant to aid you in channeling your own powerful energies. These spells do not exert power over others (spells of this type are dangerous and should be avoided at all costs) but rather work in a way to attract and magnetize positive forces from the Universe towards you. The oils connect you to the plants from which they came, the plants connect you to nature and the Universe, and the spells manifest your thoughts so that the Universe can hear them and respond.

The first one is to attract love into your life. Put a few drops of Joy on your right hand, rub it clockwise over your heart 7 times, and say out loud:

On the broom I'm flying high
Reaching, reaching to Divine
Take my wish and make it real
Make my soulmate appear!

The second one is to help you forgive someone. Put a few drops of Release on your right hand, rub it clockwise over your liver 7 times, and say out loud:

On the broom I'm flying high
Reaching, reaching to Divine

Take my wish and make it real
Make my anger disappear!

The third one is to help you to find your dream job. Put a few drops of Live Your Passion on your left hand, rub it with your right hand 7 times, and say out loud:

On the broom I'm flying high
Reaching, reaching to Divine
Take my wish and make it real
Make my perfect job appear!

The fourth one is to help you heal broken heart or remove sadness. Put a few drops of Geranium on your right hand, rub it clockwise over your heart 7 times, and say out loud:

On the broom I'm flying high
Reaching, reaching to Divine
Take my wish and make it real
Make my sorrow disappear!

The fifth one is to help you release pain. Put a few drops of Panaway where you experience discomfort (stay away from eyes), massage it in 7 times, and say out loud:

On the broom I'm flying high
Reaching, reaching to Divine
Take my wish and make it real
Make my pain disappear!

The sixth one is to bring you support in having a clear vision about your future. Put a few drops of Inspiration on your wrists, rub them together 7 times, and say out loud:

> On the broom I'm flying high
> Reaching, reaching to Divine
> Take my wish and make it real
> Make my vision very clear!

The seventh one is to bring you good luck. Put a few drops of Valor II on your wrists, rub them together 7 times, and say out loud:

> On the broom I'm flying high
> Reaching, reaching to Divine
> Take my wish and make it real
> Make good luck and joy appear!

Experiment with essential oils, but please always treat them with respect: they are living, conscious energies whose purpose is to help you heal. Thank them often, store them in a special container, and enjoy their magic!

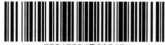

75215724R00210

Made in the USA
Middletown, DE
03 June 2018